WANT A SUREFIRE WILL QUICKLY HEL... ...U FLATTEN YOUR BELLY, SCULPT YOUR UPPER BODY, INCREASE STRENGTH AND GIVE YOU THE ARMS, UPPER BODY AND ABS YOU DESERVE – FAST?

Well, look no further.

Introducing the Revolutionary **42 Day Upper Body Fix** a simple, day-by-day breakthrough workout plan that will flatten your belly, sculpt your arms and transform your entire upper body - even if you've failed in the past.

This upper body *2-Phase blueprint* will easily fit into your busy schedule while transforming your entire upper body FASTER than anything else you have ever seen or used. *Phase 1 (21 days)* will ignite your metabolism and prime your lower body and core muscles to handle *Phase 2 (21 days)*. *Phase 2* is the most advanced phase that will help you burn all your unwanted fat, build sexy, tone muscle and give you all the amazing results you desire.

This Most Powerful Upper Body Transformation plan is guaranteed to start working within just a few days, not weeks. You will immediately start to feel it working after just a few workouts.

Image how good it will feel in just 42 days to show off tone and lean arms in your sleeveless dress, feel body confident, love your flat belly, and have others comment, " You look amazing!"

Get your copy of the **42 Day Upper Body Fix** now. This is your chance to finally get your fastest solution to transform your upper body and belly without paying thousands for a Top Trainer.

STEPS TO GET THE BEST RESULTS.

- Read Over the diet and prepare all the foods that are necessary to get started.
- Always consult with your medical professional before starting any exercise and/or diet program.
- Recommended for best results but not all needed: Purchase 4-5 sets of dumbbells ranging from 5lbs to 20 lbs, a fitness ball 55 to 60 cm, 10 to 20 lb. medicine ball, fitness mat, running or walking shoes, jump rope and a blue or red fitness band.
- Challenge yourself with heavier weights.
- Eliminate access salts, sugars, refined carbohydrates, processed foods, artificial ingredients and alcohol for the 42 days.
- Try to maintain your amazing results with a healthy lifestyle. i.e. Daily exercise and a Mediterranean Diet.

What if somedays you're short on time?

No problem. Perform just 1 to 2 circuits of that workout or simply perform an exercise from each exercise just once from each circuit and at the end perform high intensity running in place, sprinting or anything that will raise your heart rate for 2 to 5 minutes.

How to perform the workout?

Perform from top to bottom. Perform as written for best results unless short on time or medical condition. Perform all exercises and sets of each circuit before proceeding to the next circuit. Use heavier weights as you go through each circuit when applicable. Lower reps equal heavier weights (5-10 reps). Use Lighter weights when reps are high (12-30). You may also use heavy weight for the first 4-6 reps then use lighter weights to finish the set for best results.

How to get leaner and stronger?
Slowly increase the weight resistance each week. Make sure to keep good form but challenge yourself with weight that you struggle with towards the end of each exercise. Example: if you can perform curls with 10lbs. for 10 reps with little challenge, increase to 12lbs. Once it is doable perform with 15lbs.

What is most important when dieting?
Don't diet. Eat smart and healthy. Consume small meals throughout the day until satisfied but never full. Drink water all day along with an electrolyte supplement.

Eliminate refined sugars to lose weight quickly which includes alcohol. Make sure to read labels for hidden sugars. Never eat artificial sugars in any food including drinks.

Increase your lean proteins daily. Eating 3-5 ounces lean protein, 3-4x per day is satisfactory. Consume berries and greens at least 2 meals.

What if I'm dieting and working out but the weight is not showing on the scale?
Don't fret. Lift heavier, train with intensity, increase cardio and keep going. Make sure to look at your diet too, i.e. nuts and avocado 2-3x per day can slow down weight loss. Yes, they both are good fats but sometimes they can add too many calories if consumed frequently or in large quantity. I'd recommend one of each only once per day if you're are struggling. However, these foods shouldn't keep you from making progress if you are training as in the manual with intensity. Again, count your fat intake.

Will focusing just on upper body hurt progress in my lower body?

No. This workout manual has lower body workouts plus cardio. This manual is made to make a big change quickly in your upper body. Focusing on a body part that you'd like to change is ok as long as you're still training your entire body.

How do I get stronger?

Slowly increase weight pounds with each exercise overtime. This plan will not only make you stronger but will increase your cardio and muscular endurance.

Best: drop sets (perform first few reps 3-5 reps with very challenging weight i.e. 15 to 20 lbs and then pick up lighter weight to finish reps in the program i.e. 10-12lbs for 5-10 more reps.)

ARE YOU READY TO GET GOING?

Lets Go! You can do this ☺.

Start with phase 1 to increase your muscle endurance using mostly body weight exercises. Phase 2 you will add resistance with dumbbells and higher reps.

All the exercises have a picture to show the exact steps for the proper form. Exercise descriptions will tell you how to perform each exercise plus tell you what to do and not to do.

ute, sell or transmit any content written in the 42 Day Lower Body Fix without the Body studio Corp. or Doug Bennett's prior written consent. Nothing in these Terms of Use shall be interpreted as granting any license of intellectual property rights to you. This will lead to court action.

The 42 Day Upper Body Fix and/or Doug Bennett, author, writes an exact diet and workout system that can help you get amazing lower body results. However, you must use it to get your desired results. Always, consult a qualified medical professional before starting this or any other diet and fitness program. You are assuming all risk and liability by reading and using any of the material written in the The 42 Day Upper Body Fix and/or created by Douglas Bennett. Always stop if you feel discomfort and seek medical help immediately. Results are based upon each individual. Results will vary. Thus, there is no guarantee based upon every individuals certain limits, medical history, injuries or past fitness history.

EXERCISE DESCRIPTIONS:

ARMS

Push-Ups: arms, abs, core

Start in a prone position with your hands wider than shoulder width and at shoulder height. Knee position: both knees together, lean forward and drop your hips so that your head, shoulder, hips and knees are one straight line. Foot Position: place both feet together or shoulder width apart on balls of feet. Inhale and descend to 1-2 inches from floor. Squeeze your triceps and press up while exhaling. Keep navel pulled in tight and squeeze glutes throughout exercise.

Don't: place hand position above your head/keep hips higher than lower back

Do: place hand position at shoulder level/keep hips level and in line with shoulder and knees

Push-ups on knees: same as above. One long line from knees to shoulders. Keep hips down in line with body.

Power Push-ups: same as push up position. Descend and explode up off of your palms with straight arms into the air (palms go off of ground). Land back on your palms and bend elbows to decelerate. Repeat

Triangle push-ups: same as the push up but you're going to create an open triangle with your fingers. Slightly turn your hands so that your index fingers and thumbs nearly touch one another. Hands should between your face and chest and/or directly in front of your face.

Standing Curls: arms, biceps

- Start in standing with feet hip distance apart. Hold a dumbbell in each hand with palms up. Back of hand resting on each thigh.
- Curl keeping your elbows into your body while curling dumbbell straight up so it lands directly in front of each shoulder.
- Squeeze your bicep at the top and slowly lower the weight down.

Note: challenge yourself with heavier dumbbells for the first few reps and drop down in weight if needed. Example: start with 15-20lbs for 3-6 reps and then complete the set with 10-12lbs for than next 8-12 reps.

Don't: use too light of weight. Swing the weight up. Let the weight drop fast.

Do: squeeze the bicep throughout exercise. Let down the weight slowly with resistance.

CONCENTRATION CURLS:

- Sit on a bench or chair. Lean over and place hand on opposite thigh.
- Place the other arms elbow in the area interesting at the thigh and hand.
- Hang the dumbbell down with that arm and curl the dumbbell horizontally toward the shoulder.
- Squeeze the bicep on top and slowly lower.

- Use heavier weight and drop weight to increase reps. Pulse on top for extra work.

Low to High Plank: arms (triceps), core

- Start in a push up position (hands and feet on ground). Drop down on the right forearm then the left forearm (now you're in a low plank position).
- Right arm example: go up on right hand to straighten out right arm and then go up on left hand to start back up to starting position. Repeat on the right side for the set reps of plan. So, down on right forearm then left forearm, then go up on right hand and then left hand.
- Squeeze your tricep of the arm focusing on.

Don't: let hips sag or be high.

Do: keep fingers wide and straight forward. Keep hips parallel, legs locked and strong. Abs engaged entire time.

OVERHEAD TRICEP PRESS:

- Hold a dumbbell vertical over your head with one hand over the other. Don't grip the handle.
- Make sure the dumbbell is vertical when your bring it down behind your head by bending your elbows and is vertical when returning to bring dumbbell over your head (don't let the dumbbell go horizontal by bringing it up and over your head, keep it behind your head)
- Bend and extend.

PUSH BACKS:

- Hold a dumbbell in each hand.

- Lean Forward with one foot forward to support back.
- Make sure dumbbells are horizontal with palms facing up next to hip.
- Press the dumbbells back with locked arms. Press palms back until arms can't go back further and hold 2-3 seconds while squeezing triceps (back of arm).
- Return slowly and repeat
- Last rep, pulse the dumbbells 2-3 inches with arms all the way back.
- Use heavy dumbbells 10-20lbs.

Make

45 Degree Chest Press (abs, arms and chest)

- Hold a dumbbell in each hand, horizontal. Lie on back. Start with knees bent and feet in air.
- Lock out legs at 45 degrees, toes pointed.
- Engage abs at the same time as performing a chest press straight up. Lock out arms and return to repeat.
- If lower back or abs become fatigued, start over or place feet on ground while performing press on bench or floor.

Make sure the

Regular Dumbbell Curls

- Feet hip distance apart. Knees slightly bent. Hold a dumbbell in each hand horizontal. Your hands should start resting on your thigh not on the outside of your thighs at shoulder width.

- Bring the dumbbells straight up so when at top they should be right in front of your shoulder.
- Slowly Return them back to your thighs
- Pyramid your weights for better resistance, start heavy and go lighter (example : 20lbs down to 10lbs.)
- Up fast and down slow. Squeeze the bicep going up.

Tip: towards the end go half way up and back down. Half reps for added resistance. (pulsing)

Hammer Dumbbell Curls

- Feet together. Hold dumbbells vertical by your side.
- Bend elbows to curl so the dumbbells tap the front of your shoulder. Keep elbows by your side.
- Make sure your elbows aren't behind your back.
- Up fast and down slow. Squeeze the bicep going up.

Tip: towards the end go half way up and back down. Half reps for added resistance. (pulsing)

Band Curls:

- Same as the regular dumbbell curls but with a band (blue or red)
- Blue adds more resistance (recommended)
- Best after using dumbbells
- Step on the middle of the band with feet hip distance apart
- This exercise is best done quickly (burn out set)

Tip: towards the end go half way up and back down. Half reps for added resistance. (pulsing)

Tricep Bench:

- Side of SECURE bench place palms on side with fingers facing down.
- Place feet hip distance apart in front of you with feet flat, knees bent and your lower back should be skimming the bench the ENTIRE EXERCISE!
- DO NOT STRAIGHTEN YOUR LEGS IN FRONT OF YOU!! This adds pressure to the front of your shoulder and is not good!!!!
- Squeeze your tricep on top of extension.

Tip: keep feet 2-3 inches wide and place a heavy dumbbell on upper thighs (20-40lbs) so can roll off to add resistance. Make sure upper back slides ½ inch from side of bench.

MOUNTAIN CLIMBERS:

- Push up position. Feet hip distance apart. Drop hips slightly by bending elbows slightly in locked position or place hands on dumbbells etc..
- Start by driving one leg up while other stays back, both feet hit the ground (balls of feet) simultaneously! While one goes up the other goes back.
- DRIVE both balls of feet into the ground. You're going up a mountain. Don't let the front foot just dangle in the air.
- Both feet are driving into the ground. Don't let hips bounce up and down. Keep abs in tight.

BURPEES W/ PUSH UP:

- Feet hip distance apart
- Squat down and place hands by feet flat.
- Jump feet back hip width, straight leg and perform a push up
- Press up 1 inch from ground and jump feet back under you.
- Stand and repeat.

POWER PUSH UPS ON KNEES/FEET

- On knees: start with hands in front so your thumbs are in line with your arm pits and hands slightly wider than shoulder width. Elbows NOT to sides.
- Knees on ground your body should be straight line from your shoulder to your knee.
- Go down and press up in order for your hands to go off the ground, straight arm, body should be kept straight (don't bend at the hips) and return with soft elbows (not locked) and go down with resistance and push up to repeat.
- On Feet: same but you start up in regular push up position.

STRAIGHT BAR CURL

- Feet hip distance apart. Knees slightly bent. Hold a bar (15-25lb.) horizontal. Your hands should start resting on your thigh not on the outside of your thighs at shoulder width.
- Bring the bar straight up so when at top your hands should be right in front of your shoulder.
- Slowly Return them back to your thighs
- Up fast and down slow. Squeeze the bicep going up.

Tip: towards the end go half way up and back down. Half reps for added resistance. (pulsing)

BURPEES W/ 10 HIGH KNEE RUNS

- Feet hip distance apart
- Squat down and place hands by feet flat.
- Jump feet back hip width, straight leg and let upper body go down to ground
- Press up off floor using palms with arms in push up position

hard in order to land your feet under your hips to land in squat position.

- Stand and start running high knees
- 10 High Knees you will bring up each knee/foot 10x.
- Running high knee on balls of feet
- Drive knees up hip height
- Opposite hand drives up with opposite knee
- Keep abs tight. Think of driving elbows up and back in locked bent position.

BURPEES W/ PUSH UP TO A STAR:

- Feet hip distance apart
- Squat down and place hands by feet flat.
- Jump feet back hip width, straight leg and let upper body go down to ground
- Press up off floor using palms with arms in push up position hard in order to land your feet under your hips to land in squat position
- Now stand up and perform a star

KICK BACKS BAND (BLUE OR RED):

- Wrap band around a secure post or stand on one side for tension.
- Hold handle with palm up and lean over with opposite leg forward and place hand without band on your front knee or place hand on secure platform for stability.
- Draw elbow high and tight to your side that's holding handle. Make sure elbow is higher than your hand for more tension.
- Pull back on band for tension. Know straighten arm keeping elbow tight to side.
- Squeeze tricep on top position and slowly bring back to bent

position (just greater than 90 degrees to keep tension on tricep entire exercise)

Tip: extend and bend inch only and pulse your reps at the very end of the exercise for burn.

SHOULDERS:

SHOULDER PRESS:

- Feet hip distance apart. Hold a dumbbell in each hand (start light!). Palms facing out or towards your ears (vertical).
- Inhale and exhale to press straight up overhead. Lock out elbows on top.
- DON'T bring the weights together overhead as this works your neck not shoulders.
- Challenge yourself but if you begin to fail to press up half way overhead, stop immediately as pressing through can hurt your shoulder.

Tips: vary hand position every other reps, horizontal and vertical. Perform drop sets (start with heavy and go lighter as reps increase, i.e. start with 15lbs for 3-4 reps and drop to 10lbs immediately for 5-8 more reps). Pulse the weight when extended overhead in the last reps.

SIDE RAISES:

- Feet hip distance apart. Hold dumbbell in each hand by your side.
- Raise straight out and away to shoulder height.

- Once as shoulder height, hold 2 seconds and let down slowly to resist gravity.

BENT OVER RAISES:

- Sitting or standing. Lean over and place dumbbells directly under you and in front of your face with slightly bent but locked arms.
- Use your back upper back and shoulder muscles to bring dumbbells up and out. Squeezing shoulder blades once on top.
- Hold 2 seconds while squeezing upper back muscles and let down slow.

BACK

ONE ARM ROWS:

- Place one knee and hand on a bench or place your hand on a support at hip height and keep feet hip distance apart and lean forward.
- Pull the dumbbell up high with elbow in to your side. Elbow should be higher than back once you're on top.
- Hold up 2-3 seconds and squeeze upper back. Let down slow and repeat.

LEGS

Squat: glutes, hamstrings, quads

- Start with your feet slightly greater than hip distance apart and toes turned out slightly. Squat below parallel while driving hips back and shoulders slightly forward.
- Drive up on HEELs and engage glutes to return to the starting position.

AIR SQUATS:

While squatting down bring arms straight up and out at eye level. Bring back to hip level while standing.

Don't: lean forward to place pressure on your knee cap/ lean over while squatting/ bounce on bottom/

Do: go 1-2 inches below parallel/drive thru your heels. When at top, drive hips forward to engage glutes while standing.

With Medicine Ball: hold ball with fingers facing up and palms under ball.

With dumbbell: hold dumbbell parallel (with one hand on each end, palm up under your chin) or vertical (goblet squat). NOTE: goblet squat best for a deeper vertical squat that targets your inner thighs and glutes.

Medical warning: do not perform with a knee, leg, and groin or calf injury. Consult doctor first.

Lunges: glutes, hamstrings, quads

- Start with feet hip distance apart. Hands behind head, holding dumbbells or on waist. Keep shoulders back while stepping one foot forward landing on front heel. Back leg should create a 90 degree angle to floor.
- Drive off front heel forcefully so that front toe comes off the ground and feet land back to hip distance apart.

Lunge Pulses: glutes, hamstrings, quads

Start with feet hip distance apart. Hands behind head, holding dumbbells or on waist. Keep shoulders back while stepping one foot forward landing on front heel. Back leg should create a 90 degree angle to floor. Now, instead of driving off your front foot to stand back up straight, stay in the lunge position and pulse your back knee up and down 2-4 inches from the ground for the time in program.

Walking lunge: same as the stationary lunges. Difference: you're stepping into a lunge while walking.

- Start with your feet hip distance apart and step forward into a lunge. Once your front foot hits the ground the back knee should drop down as above.
- Bring back foot next to front and repeat with the other leg.

Don't: let your front knee go beyond front toe

Do: make sure back leg is bent 90 degrees (if not then step closer or further out). Make sure feet are hip distance entire time of exercise.

Medical warning: do not perform with a knee, groin, leg or calf injury. Consult doctor first.

Reverse Lunge with Kick: glutes, hamstrings, quads

- Start with feet hip distance apart while holding a dumbbell in each hand (5-20lbs). Step back into a lunge and bring your back foot knee back to front and up high (hip height) to snap the foot forward in a kicking position.
- After kicking that foot bring it down and back to a lunge with the same foot. Repeat on one side until all reps performed.

Please note that the wrong form will lead to a possible injured lower back, tight hip flexors, strained neck muscles and little results. Place your feet under a sturdy support or free form. Keep feet hip distance apart and 4-6 inches from your glutes (bent knees).

Don't: bring your back leg straight up from behind to kick. Make sure to bring your knee up in front and snap your kick out.

Do: use a challenging weight in each hand. Snap your kicks out in front.

Star Jumps: glutes, hamstring, quads, cardio

- Start in a tucked position as if downhill skiing (feet together, lean forward, arms pulled in, bent knees). Explode off your legs and straighten your arms and legs out wide while in the air.
- Bring feet back together before hitting the ground.
- Once you hit the ground go back into a tucked position.

Jumping Squat: glutes, hamstrings, quads, cardio

Option 1: Start with feet hip distance apart and hands facing your ears. Squat down, shoot your arms straight up toward ceiling while exploding off the ground using the energy obtained from squatting.

Option 2: feet together, squat straight down so your balls of feet on ground and heels off the ground. Your bum should almost hit your heels. Jump straight up high. Land back on both feet and slow squat down to explode back up.

Don't: explode off the ground and land into a squat.

Do: explode up and land onto both feet and start again. Don't jump into a squat.

With dumbbell: hold dumbbell parallel (with one hand on each end, palm up under your chin) or hold a dumbbell in each hand, arms straight by your sides. Use option 1 for legs.

With medicine ball: hold medicine ball (10-20lbs) with palms facing up to chest and under chin entire time. Squat below parallel and explode up as high as you can. Once you hit the ground, pause 1 sec and repeat. Don't jump from one jumping squat to the other. **ALWAYS RESET.**

Good Mornings: legs (hamstrings), glutes

- Feet hip distance apart and heels slightly elevated (1 inch) off floor with a support (dumbbell handle). Hold a dumbbell in each hand (palms facing body).
- Shoulders back, arms locked and straight. Slowly lean down and forward with dumbbells towards instep of foot. Keep shoulders back and head straight.
- Squeeze glutes and engage hamstrings to bring weight and shoulders back to returning position (upright).

Back Leg Curl with ball: legs (hamstrings), glutes

- Lie in supine position with your feet up on a physio ball. Place heals on midpoint on top of ball. Flex toes toward you. Lock knees out.
- Keep hips off ground and engage your abs plus glutes. Pull the ball to you with heels. Keep your toes toward you the whole time.
- Roll the ball back out while keeping your hips level and off the ground creating one long line from heel to shoulder.

Power tip: place arms straight up toward ceiling during entire exercise.

Don't: drop hips while rolling ball to or away from you/ squeeze glutes throughout exercise

Do: keep toes flexed/ emphasize hamstrings and glutes to pull ball to you/keep knees high when pulling the ball to you.

Stand Ups: legs (quads), glutes (bum)

- Start standing with feet hip distance apart. Right leg example: reverse lunge down to right knee on mat. Then drop down the left knee.
- Now step straight up with right foot so you're in a lunge position (right foot on ground, left knee still on ground).
- Push off the right foot to stand up and repeat by dropping the right knee and then the left knee.

Don't: step out to the side or close.

Do; step straight out and in front of your body as if lunging straight out. Make sure all pressure is pushing off the front heel to stand up.

Split Squat (jumping lunges):

- Spring up off ground with both feet at hip distance apart splitting your legs into a lunge position and landing in a stationary lunge position on the balls of your feet.
- Once your toes hit the ground bend both knees and go down until your back knee is 1 inch from the ground.
- Engage your butt and legs and bound straight back up to a straight leg position off the ground. Switch legs in the air and repeat.

Don't: land on the front foot so that the front knee goes beyond the front toe/ land with legs straight and knees locked/ keep back leg straight

Do: jump with power off your toes/get into rhythm and land in the same correct position at all times/ let back knee bend till 1-2 inches from ground/ start out slow to get rhythm / Explode with force by engaging glutes, quads and calves.

Medical warning: do not perform with a knee, heart, groin, leg or calf injury. Consult doctor.

Skating: glutes, quads, cardio

- Feet together. Squat and lean over.
- Push off the right SIDE OF FOOT (HEEL) to jump to the left and land on left foot while bring right ball of foot over to the left foot.
- Now push off the left SIDE OF FOOT (HEEL, NOT TOE) to jump to the right and land right foot while bringing left ball of foot over to the right foot.
- Repeat back and forth.

Tips: don't bring back foot behind like a curtsy. Make sure to lean over entire time and squat. Focus on bum, cardio and quads. Don't spring up. Think of going lateral while staying squat and forward.

Hip Raises with/without dumbbell: glutes, hamstrings

- Start in a supine position (lying on back) with knees bent and feet on ground 2-4 inches from your glutes. Point feet slightly turned out.
- Hold medicine ball or dumbbell on your pelvis with both hands. Engage glutes, pull in navel and press off ground with heels.
- Raise pelvis squeezing your glutes tightly for 2 seconds. Return slowly to the mat. Repeat.

Don't: press off toes/ place feet more than 4 inches from glutes/ use arms to raise ball

Do: ball should be kept centered on pelvis throughout exercise not at your navel

Single leg Hip Raise: glute, hamstring

- Perform this exercise exactly as done with hip raises with ball but only use one leg. Keep your heel in straight line with middle of glute that's on the same side as foot.
- Raise the other foot to ceiling with toe flexed toward you.

Plie' squat Pulses: glutes, inner thighs, quads

- Place feet slightly greater than hip distance apart and turn toes out. Squat down 1 inch from parallel. Your back should be straight, navel engaged, shoulders back.
- Pulse (lower and raise 2-3 inches from the lowest position)

while holding low squat position. Hand position on top of thighs, on hips or behind head.

Don't: keep feet narrow/ bring shoulders forward/ emphasize toes

Do: squeeze your glutes throughout entire exercise/Keep navel in/ press into heels

Plie' squat: glutes, inner thighs, quads

- Place feet slightly greater than hip distance apart and turn toes out. Place palms of hands high up on thighs, behind head or on hips and press down on thighs to create pressure on legs.
- Squat down 1 inch from parallel.
- Your back should be straight, navel engaged, shoulders back.

Don't: keep feet narrow/ bring shoulders forward/ emphasize toes

Do: squeeze your glutes throughout entire exercise/Keep navel in/ press into heels

Plie' Squat with Dumbbell: same as above but hold a dumbbell vertical. The heavier the better.

Tip: place both feet on a platform (benches, boxes or stacked weighted plates) that are 4-6 inches off the ground so you can dip low without the vertical dumbbell hitting the ground which allows you to get deeper with you squat.

Kettle Bell or Dumbbell Swings: 2 ways:

Best way:

- **hold a dumbbell between legs and lean forward in order to thrust hips forward to get the kettle bell or dumbbell to swing forward.
- As the weight of the kettlebell or dumbbell swings back your hips will follow.

Second Swing:

- Start in squat position with back up straight and hips lowered in squat position with weight hanging between legs (straight arm).
- Now, to start you'll use the momentum from straightening up into standing position (throw your hips forward and squeeze your glutes on top) with the weight going up until eye level 3-4 inches above your head.
- As the weight descends with straight arms, you'll go back to quatting position. Repeat for allotted time.

** HOLD THE DUMBBELL HANDLE WITH BOTH HANDS SO THE DUMBBELL IS VERTICAL.

Burpees: cardio, quads, hamstrings, calves, arms, abs

Warning: never perform with a knee or back injury. Replace all burpees with a star jump.

- Start in a standing position with feet hip distance apart. Hands by your side.
- Begin by bending at the legs with your back straight and head up. Place hands down on ground by your feet and begin to throw your feet back while placing your weight onto your palms.
- Land on the balls of your feet with knees slightly bent. Let your entire body rest on the ground and press hard off the palms of your hands so your upper body pushes up off the ground while your feet jump up under your hips hip distance apart into a squat position. Now, return into standing position. Repeat

Don't: Arch back while throwing your feet back into parallel position/ bend back and look down to bring your hands onto the ground/ throw your feet back wider than hip distance apart.

Do: perform exercise in a steady and safe manner/ stand up completely before repeating exercise/ keep hips slightly raises while in parallel position to protect lower back

Burpees with Jump: same as above. Yet, when returning to standup position begin to explode off of toes with power and straighten legs while pointing toes in the air. Return to the ground softly and with a soft landing by bending knees.

Burpees with dumbbells: same as above but hold a dumbbell in each hand. Place the dumbbell on the ground as above and stand up with dumbbells. Best to use 8 – 15lbs.

Burpees with Mountain climbers: same as above. Yet, your will stay in a push up (parallel) position and perform mountain climbers.

Do: keep your body in boxing position (shoulder facing opponent)/ utilize your obliques/ keep elbows tucked into body throughout exercise/ optional: bend right knee while slipping to right and vice versa.

Calf Raises: calves

Place balls of feet onto a step or edge of box. Raise the heels up and down to work your calves.

Set 1:
Feet parallel: Feet straight and hip distance apart for parallel position.

Set 2:
Toes out, Heels Together: place balls of feet wide on edge and heels together off the edge. Bring heels up and down for calve raises.

Set 3:
Toes in, Heels Out: place balls of feet in and on edge. Heels out wide off the edge. Brings heels up and down for calve raises.

Quad Blaster: legs (quads), calves

- Hold onto a railing or a firm support. Bring your feet 4-5 inches from the support. Feet should be hip distance apart. Grab the support and lean back so that your arms are straight and elbows are locked out. Go up onto the balls of your feet and keep heels up the entire exercise.
- Squat down until your bottom almost touches your heels and then come back up till your quads are at a 90 degree angle to your shins. Go back down and repeat. Shaking legs is normal.

Back N' Forth: legs, calves, cardio

- Start to the right of a 15-20 foot line (hips parallel to the line), feet together.

- Stay on the balls of feet. Hands behind head.
- Jump right to left 1 inch from the line or over a cone and left to right.

HIGH KNEE RUNS:

- Running high knee on balls of feet
- Drive knees up hip height
- Opposite hand drives up with opposite knee
- Keep abs tight. Think of driving elbows up and back in locked bent position.

ABS

POWER PUSH UPS:

On knees: start with hands in front so your thumbs are in line with your arm pits and hands slightly wider than shoulder width. Elbows NOT to sides.

- Knees on ground your body should be straight line from your shoulder to your knee.
- Go down and press up in order for your hands to go off the ground, straight arm, body should be kept straight (don't bend at the hips) and return with soft elbows (not locked) and go down with resistance and push up to repeat.

On Feet: same but you start up in regular push up position. Feet wide.

HIGH PLANK WALKING:

- Same as high plank but walking feet. Get into push up position with feet hip distance and on toes, straight leg and body one long line from shoulder to heel.
- Hands slightly wider than shoulder width, fingers open and straight with pressure on palms slightly under shoulder so thumbs in line with arm pits.
- Suck in navel entire time
- Inhale and exhale with each foot that rises and bring up navel tighter and tighter.
- Foot flexed and heels pushed back squeeze glute that lifts that leg. Leg straight push back on heel entire time (don't point toe) keep tension on glute and lift right leg. Squeeze on top and return to ground and lift leg same.
- Repeat lifting alternate feet entire exercise keeping stomach in and engaging bum.

X-LEG CRUNCHES:

- Lie on your back. Fingers behind ears pressing into skull for support. Flex chest up to engage stomach a little before exercise starts with shoulder blades slightly off the ground, chin 1 inch from chest.
- X Ankles and keep knees shoulder width the entire time and knees slightly forward to engage your lower abs (keep feet up knee level, don't let them drop)
- Crunch higher by inhaling and exhaling through pursed lips, Hold on top.
- Return to crunch position. DON'T let your head go back. STAY in crunch position and keep tension on abs entire time.
- Make each crunch tighter.

Tip: pulse on top for small crunches to put extra emphasis on abs at end of exercise.

MOUNTAIN CLIMBERS:

- Push up position. Feet hip distance apart. Drop hips slightly by bending elbows slightly in locked position or place hands on dumbbells etc..
- Start by driving one leg up while other stays back, both feet hit the ground (balls of feet) simultaneously! While one goes up the other goes back.
- DRIVE both balls of feet into the ground. You're going up a mountain. Don't let the front foot just dangle in the air.
- Both feet are driving into the ground. Don't let hips bounce up and down. Keep abs in tight.

BICYCLE:

- Start in a crunch position with knees bent and at 90 degrees to floor with toes pointed away from your head. Keep Elbows wide, slightly forward and locked in position.
- Initiate by extending your left leg out, bring right knee up while keeping your elbows wide and twisting your left elbow and shoulder in direction of right knee.
- Keep your upper body flexed throughout entire exercise in crunch position. Perform at a steady slow pace. Imagine placing your back flat up against a board and you should twist one side of your body in one motion. Act as if you are reaching opposite shoulder to opposite knee.
- Legs should pass one another in the center as there is an imaginary line dividing your body in two halves

Leg Flutter:

- Place hands under your glutes for lower back support. Advanced: start with crunch position (hands behind ears) and keep pelvis neutral position (level).
- Start with bent knees and inhale as you kick legs straight out 3-6 inches off the ground with STRAIGHT TOES, LOCKED OUT KNEES AS IF laser beams are shooting out of your toes the ENTIRE TIME!
- Squeeze quads, lock out knees, straight feet now flutter one foot pass the other 3-4 inches.

Kick outs:

- Place hands under your glutes for lower back support. Advanced: start with crunch position (hands behind ears) and keep pelvis neutral position (level).
- Start with bent knees (table top position, toes pointed) and inhale as you kick legs straight out 3-6 inches off the ground with STRAIGHT TOES, LOCKED OUT KNEES AS IF laser beams are shooting out of your toes the ENTIRE TIME!
- Now return to bent position and repeat

Knee Tucks:

- Start on your back with arms overhead and palms facing each other. Hands 2-3 inches from ground.
- Legs straight out or wide but knees locked out, toes pointed.
- As you sit up simultaneously draw knees up to your chest and wrap arms around knees. As you roll back, kick your arms and legs out to beginning position and repeat.

VARIATIONS:

- Don't allow arms and legs to touch ground.
- Shoot out arms and legs wide when laying out to represent a star position and tuck all in when sitting up.

ABS

Plank: core, thighs, shoulders

- Get in a prone position on your forearms and toes.
- Keep your body in one long line from your heel to your shoulder.
- Slightly elevate your hips if you have a weak core or back injury. Forearms should be directly under your shoulders and upper body.
- Feet together or out wide for advanced, navel pulled in and glutes tight.

Plank on ball is same position but with forearms on balance ball. Roll elbows away from you with the ball 2-4 inches and roll back.

High Plank: same as plank position but you're elevated on your palms as in a push up position. Fingers straight forward and palms directly under shoulder with elbows locked.

Walking in plank or high plank: in plank position squeeze your glute tightly and raise one flexed foot at a time off the ground 2-3 inches. Switch feet back and forth.

Don't: let your hips go below a straight line/Bend knees/keep elbows away from the shoulders

Do: keep one long line/tighten glutes / pull navel up

Leg Raises, 90 to 3 "(vary It up with variations below):

- Lie on back. Place hands (palm down in a triangle shape) under your glutes and lower back.
- Head down and bend knees up so your shins are horizontal to ground and 90 degrees to thighs. Toes pointed. Straighten your legs and lock out knees with feet pointed 3 inches off ground.
- Make sure legs very straight and knees locked out! Abs in tight. Option: bring head up as you kick your feet out. Keep head up the entire exercise but be careful of neck strain. Keep chin down and eyes look at feet not ceiling.

Variations: Make sure feet are pointed, knees locked out and legs straight! Back never arched. Head up (optional)

1. **Flutter:** while feet are 3-6 inches off the ground, flutter your feet up and down (straight legs, feet pointed!) about 2-4 inches. You can also flutter your feet up and down as your bring your legs up to 90 degrees and then back to 3 inches off ground.

2. **Criss Cross:** while feet are 3 inches off the ground, criss cross your feet over and under each other.

3. **Wide:** while feet are 3 inches off the ground, separate your feet 3-5 inches and then return them together and repeat.

You can also hold them while they are open for 10-30 seconds.

4. **Circle Feet:** While feet are 3-6 inches off the ground, start with feet tight together and pointed away with knees locked, legs straight! Now draw a circle (6 inch diameter) with your toes going up and around. After performing 5-10 reps repeat now going the opposite direction going down and around. Always bring the toes back together.

Bicycle (abs:lower,upper)

- Lie flat in a supine position (on back). Start in a crunched position with hands lightly on head (do not lock fingers, best to place fingers on skull right behind ears), elbows wide, knees bend with shins parallel to the floor and feet pointed away from you.
- Twist your abs by turning your right elbow, shoulder and rib cage toward the left knee while simultaneously kicking your right leg straight out at 45 degrees.
- Go back to neutral and repeat the same on the left side. Repeat back and forth with a crisp and fast pace without losing form or compromising your back.

Side Plank core, obliques

Right Side Example:

- Lie on your side with your Right forearm on the ground 90 degrees to your chest. Make sure your right shoulder is aligned up with your right elbow. Right foot on the ground and your left foot resting on top.
- Keep your body in a straight line from your top ankle to top shoulder. Pretend your body is in a toaster and you've got to

keep straight up and down without getting burned. Lift your bottom hip and side up by engaging your bottom obliques. Raise top arm straight up towards ceiling with palm facing forward.

- Hold the position for the specified amount of time.

Beginners: split your feet so your bottom leg is on the ground and your top leg is bent behind the front one with foot flat on the ground for support.

VARIATION:

- Advanced: place your bottom hand down in under your shoulder rather than your forearm directly under your shoulder.
- Raise your top leg up 6-12 inches and hold.

Sit Ups: abs

- Please note that the wrong form will lead to a possible injured lower back, tight hip flexors, strained neck muscles and little results. Place your feet under a sturdy support or free form. Keep feet hip distance apart and 4-6 inches from your glutes (bent knees).
- Begin in a crunch position (chest flexed, lower shoulder blade on mat, finger tips behind ears, abs engaged and elbows wide and slightly angled towards midline). Inhale and exhale as you ascend up. Crunch up and start to roll down one vertebra at a time.
- STOP when your lower part of shoulder blade touches the mat. Stay in crunch position. Repeat. If you can't perform a full sit up then place arms out wide with palms facing up and scoop hands up into air as you excel upward and bring arms back in while going back to the mat.

Don't: pull on head/flatten out on bottom (don't allow top of shoulder blades to touch the mat) /bounce off ground

Do: go up controlled and go down with resistance utilizing ab muscles/ look over knees entire time.

Cross/Cross Sit Ups: at the top position you will twist your elbows wide right and left while keeping your ribs long (sitting up tall). Once going right and left, Slowly lower back to crunch position. Repeat.

Cross Over Taps: abs

- Start on your back with both arms and legs straight and wide. Place your right arm out to the side (90 degrees to your body) with palm down.
- Push off the hand in order to sit up to reach the left hand to the right foot across.

Don't: just reach the hand to the opposite foot.

Do: make sure you push off the hand on the ground to help you bring the opposite shoulder off the ground so your opposite hand touches the opposite foot.

45 Degree Crunches: abs

Note: follow exactly as below.

Start on your back with fingers behind your ears. Heels on ground and crunch up. Eyes looking over bent knees. Stay crunched and engage abs entire time. Bring right foot off the ground so your knee is bent in table top position (right knee parallel to the floor). Keeping in crunch (hands behind ears, chin inch from the ground, abs tight) bring left knee same. Now, point toes away. Kick both legs straight out 45 degrees from the ground and knees locked. Make sure you didn't lose the engaged abs (crunched). While legs locked, toes pointed, legs 45 degrees to the ground start doing small pulse crunches.

Once you start to feel your lower back or abs fail. Stop and start over.

Don't: stick legs out right away. First engage abs and bring legs off ground one at a time. Don't leg knees stay bent.

Do: legs should be straight out, knees locked, toes pointed like a laser beam.

Body Reboot
transformation series

Lean Arms & Flat Abs

Phase I

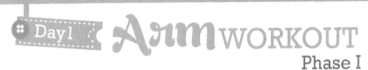

Body Reboot Transformations

Day 1 · Arm WORKOUT
Phase I

Circuit 1
Perform Exercises 1 to 3, Repeat 3x   No Rest

Jump Rope or Jumping Jacks
set 1: 1 min   set 2: 2 min   set 3: 3 min

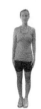
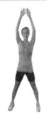
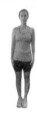

Regular Push Ups (knees)
Set 1: 10   Set 2: 15   Set 3: 20

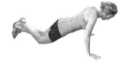
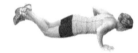
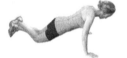

Jumping Squats
Set 1: 10   Set 2: 20   Set 3: 30

Circuit 2
Perform Exercises 1 to 3   Repeat 3x Total.   No Rest

Run High Knee
Set 1: 1 min   Set 2: 1 min   Set 3: 1 min

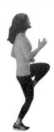

Punch Up High (with 2-3lbs dbs)   Set 1: 30 sec   Set 2: 30 sec   Set 3: 30 sec

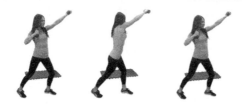

Burpees   Set 1: 10   Set 2: 20   Set 3: 30

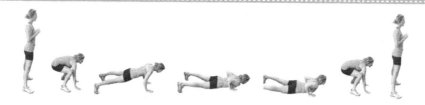

Circuit 3   Perform Exercises 1 to 3   Repeat 3x Total.   No Rest

Skating   Set 1: 1 min   Set 2: 1 min   Set 3: 1 min

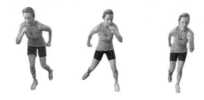

Low To High Plank (each Arm)   Set 1: 15-20   Set 2: 15   Set 3: 10

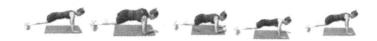

Mountain Climbers   Set 1: 1 min   Set 2: 1 min   Set 3: 1 min

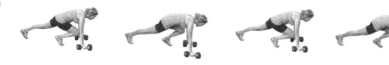

Body Reboot Transformations

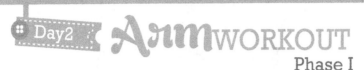

Day2 **Arm**WORKOUT

Phase I

Cardio

- Jog or Power Walk   2-3 miles

Circuit 1   Perform Each Exercises 1 to 4   Repeat 3x   No Rest

Sit Ups   Set 1: 1 min   Set 2: 1 min   Set 3: 1 min

Knee Tucks   Set 1: 25   Set 2: 25   Set 3: 25

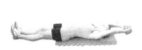
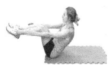
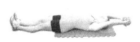

Bicycle   Set 1: 30 sec   Set 2: 30 sec   Set 3: 30 sec

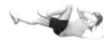
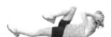

Plank   Set 1: 1 min   Set 2: 1 min   Set 3: 1 min

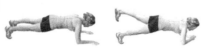
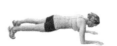

Circuit 2

Perform Each Exercises 1 to 3 Repeat 4x No Rest

Shoulder Press (Dumbbells)   Set 1: 12   Set 2: 12   Set 3: 8   Set 4: 8

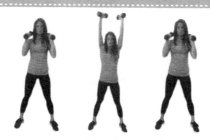

Side Raises (Dumbbells)   Set 1: 10   Set 2: 10   Set 3: 10   Set 4: 8

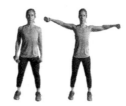

Bent Over Raises (Dumbbells)   Set 1: 15   Set 2: 15   Set 3: 12   Set 4: 12

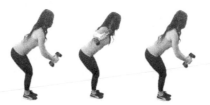

Body Reboot Transformations

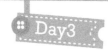 Day3 Arm WORKOUT

Phase I

Jog 1 mile

Stretch 5 to 10 minutes (hamstring, quads, calves, lower and upper back)
Sprints @ 80% max (not full sprint), 3 x 25 yards or 3 x 15 sec on treadmill
Sprints @ 80% max, 5 x 50 yards or 5 x 30 sec on treadmill

*Rest 30 sec to 1 minute between sprints depending on fitness level. If you are a beginner
simply trot at 50% max. Don't sprint!

Circuit 1 Perform Exercises 1 to 4 Repeat 4x Total No Rest

Jump Rope or Jumping Jacks with a Fist   Set 1: 1 min   Set 2: 2 min   Set 3: 2 min

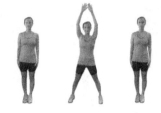

High Knee Running   Set 1: 1 min   Set 2: 1 min   Set 3: 1 min

Back N Forth   Set 1: 1 min   Set 2: 1 min   Set 3: 1 min

Burpees   Set 1: 10   Set 2: 10   Set 3: 10

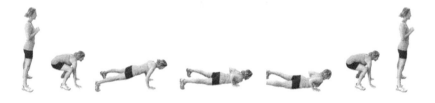

Circuit 2 Perform Exercise 1 to 5 Repeat 3x Total No Rest

Standing Curls (dumbbells)   Set 1: 10   Set 2: 10   Set 3: 10

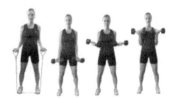

Hammer Curls (dumbbells)   Set 1: 10   Set 2: 20   Set 3: 30

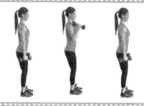

Overhead Tricep Extensions   Set 1: 20   Set 2: 20   Set 3: 20

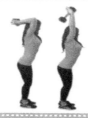

Tricep Push Ups (knees)   Set 1: 10   Set 2: 10-20   Set 3: 10-20

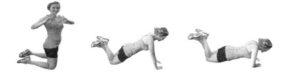

Tricep Bench Dips   Set 1: 20   Set 2: 30   Set 3: 30

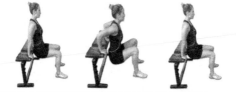

Cardio

Jog 1 mile

Body Reboot Transformations

 Day4   Arm WORKOUT

Phase I

Cardio 30 minutes

Circuit 1   Perform Exercises 1 to 3 Repeat 3x Total No Rest

Knee Tucks   Set 1: 25   Set 2: 50   Set 3: 50

 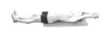

Sit Ups w twist   Set 1: 25   Set 2: 25   Set 3: 25

 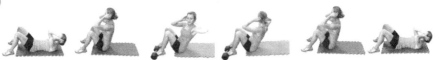

leg flutters   Set 1: 1 min   Set 2: 30 sec - 1 min   Set 3: 30 sec

 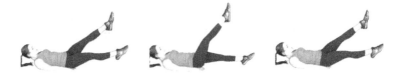

Circuit 2   Perform Exercises 1 to 3, Repeat 4x No Rest

Stand Ups (each leg)   Set 1: 20   Set 2: 20   Set 3: 20   Set 4: 10

Star Jumps   Set 1: 25 Set 2: 50 Set 3: 50 Set 4: 25

One arm Row   Set 1: 15   Set 2: 12   Set 3: 12   Set 4: 8

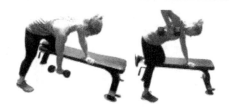

Body Reboot Transformations

Day5   ARMWORKOUT
Phase I

Jog or Power Walk 3-5 miles

Body Reboot Transformations

Day6   ARMWORKOUT
Phase I

Circuit 1   Perform Exercises 1 to 4, Repeat 4x No Rest

Jump Rope or Jumping Jacks with a Fist   Set 1: 1 min   Set 2: 2 min   Set 3: 2 min   Set 4: 2 min

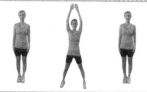

Standing Curls   Set 1: 25   Set 2: 15   Set 3: 10   Set 4: 10

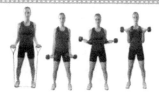

45 Degree Chest Press   Set 1: 12   Set 2: 12   Set 3: 12   Set 4: 8

 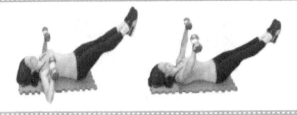

Regular Push Ups   Set 1: 15-20   Set 2: 25-30   Set 3: 25-50   Set 4: 15-20

 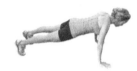 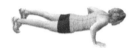 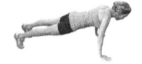

Circuit 2   Perform Exercises 1 to 4, Repeat 3x No Rest

Mountain Climbers   Set 1: 1 min   Set 2: 1 min   Set 3: 1 min

    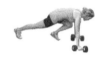

Hammer Curls   Set 1: 25   Set 2: 25   Set 3: 25

 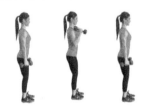

Concentration Curls   Set 1: 15   Set 2: 12   Set 3: 8-12

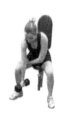 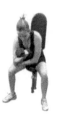 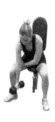

Push Ups Pulses Set 1: 25 Set 2: 25 Set 3: 25

4

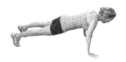 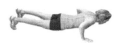 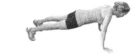

Circuit 3 Perform Exercises 1 to 3, Repeat 3x No Rest

Hip Raises Set 1: 50 Set 2: 50-100 Set 3: 50-100

1

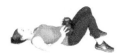 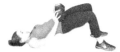 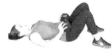

Good Mornings Set 1: 12 Set 2: 12 Set 3: 12

2

Back leg Curl (ball) Set 1: 20 Set 2: 20-30 Set 3: 20-30

3

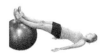 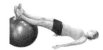

Body Reboot Transformations

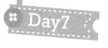 Day 7 — Arm WORKOUT

Phase I

Cardio 45-90 minutes

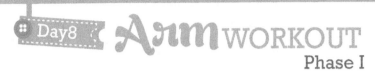

:: Day8 :: Arm WORKOUT

Phase I

Cardio 45-90 minutes

Circuit 1
Perform Exercises 1 to 4, Repeat 3x No Rest

Jump Rope or Jumping Jacks   set 1: 1 min   set 2: 2 min   set 3: 3 min

 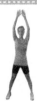

Regular Push Ups (knees)   Set 1: 10   Set 2: 20   Set 3: 20

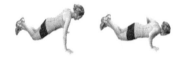

Triangle Push Ups (knees)   Set 1: 10   Set 2: 10   Set 3: 10

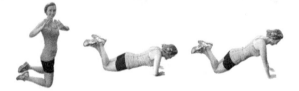

Jumping Squats   Set 1: 25   Set 2: 25   Set 3: 30

Circuit 2
Perform Exercises 1 to 4, Repeat 4x No Rest

Run High Knee   Set 1: 1 min   Set 2: 1 min   Set 4: 1 min

Punch Up High (with 2-3lbs dbs)   Set 1: 30 sec   Set 2: 30 sec   set 4: 30 sec

 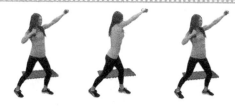

Burpees w a jump   Set 1: 10   Set 2: 25   Set 4: 25

 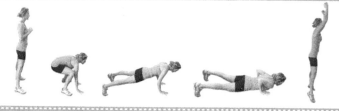

Star Jumps   Set 1: 25   Set 2: 25   Set 4: 50

  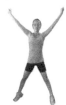

Circuit 3
Perform Exercises 1 to 4, Repeat 3x No Rest

Skating   Set 1: 1 min   Set 2: 2 min   Set 3: 2 min

  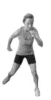

Low To High Plank (each Arm) Set 1: 15-20   Set 2: 15-20   Set 3: 15-20

2

Mountain Climbers Set 1: 1 min   Set 2: 1 min   Set 3: 1 min

3

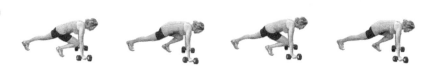

Plank with walking Set 1: 1 min   Set 2: 30 sec   Set 3: 30 sec

4

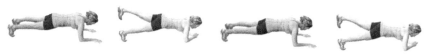

Body Reboot Transformations

Day9 Arm WORKOUT

Phase I

Jog or Power Walk 2-3 miles

Circuit 1 Perform Exercises 1 to 5, Repeat 3x No Rest

Sit Ups Set 1: 1 min   Set 2: 1 min   Set 3: 1 min

1

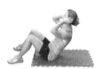

Knee Tucks   Set 1: 25   Set 2: 50   Set 3: 50

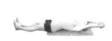 

Bicycle   Set 1: 30 sec   Set 2: 1 min   Set 3: 1 min

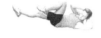 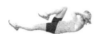

Plank   Set 1: 1 min   Set 2: 1 min   Set 3: 1-2 min

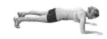

leg Raises   Set 1: 15-25   Set 2: 15-25   Set 3: 15-25

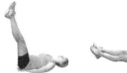 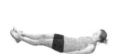

Circuit 2   Perform Exercises 1 to 4, Repeat 4x No Rest

Shoulder Press (Dumbbells)   Set 1: 12   Set 2: 12   Set 3: 8   Set 4: 8

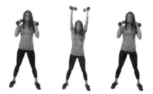

Side Raises (Dumbbells)   Set 1: 10   Set 2: 10   Set 3: 10   Set 4: 8

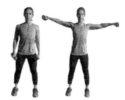

Bent Over Raises (Dumbbells) Set 1: 15   Set 2: 15   Set 3: 12   Set 4: 12

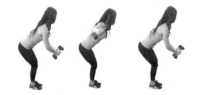

Burpees with Dumbbells   Set 1: 10   Set 2: 10   Set 3: 10   Set 4: 5

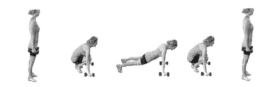

Body Reboot Transformations

Day 10 : Arm WORKOUT
Phase I

Jog 1 mile

Stretch 5 to 10 minutes (hamstring, quads, calves, lower and upper back)
Sprints @ 80% max (not full sprint), 3 x 25 yards or 3 x 15 sec on treadmill
Sprints @ 80% max, 5 x 50 yards or 5 x 30 sec on treadmill
Sprints@ 100 % max, 2 x 100 yards or 2 x 1 minute on treadmill

*rest 30 sec to 1 minute between sprints depending on fitness level. If you are a beginner
simply trot at 50% max. Don't sprint!

Circuit 1   Perform Exercises 1 to 4, Repeat 4x No Rest

Jump Rope or Jumping Jacks with a Fist   Set 1: 1 min   Set 2: 2 min   Set 3: 2 min

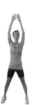

High Knee Running Set 1: 1 min   Set 2: 1 min   Set 3: 1 min

Back N Forth Set 1: 1 min   Set 2: 1 min   Set 3: 1 min

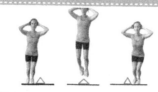

Skating Set 1: 1 min   Set 2: 1 min   Set 3: 1 min

Circuit 2 Perform Exercises 1 to 6, Repeat 3x No Rest

Standing Curls (dumbbells) Set 1: 10   Set 2: 10   Set 3: 10

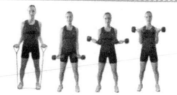

Standing Curls (dumbbells, heavier) Set 1: 5-10   Set 2: 5-10   Set 3: 5-10

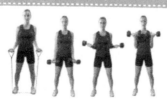

I.E. First Set of Standing Curls use 10lb dumbbells. Second Set of Standing Curls use 15 to 20 lbs.

Hammer Curls (dumbbells) Set 1: 10   Set 2: 20   Set 3: 30

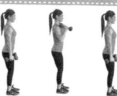

Overhead Tricep Extensions   Set 1: 20   Set 2: 20   Set 3: 20

Tricep Push Backs   Set 1: 15   Set 2: 15-20   Set 3: 15-20

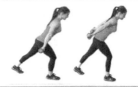

Tricep Bench Dips   Set 1: 20   Set 2: 30   Set 3: 30

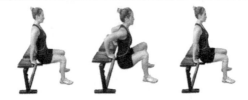

Cardio

Jog 1 mile

Body Reboot Transformations

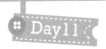 Day 1

ARmWORKOUT
Phase I

Cardio 30 minutes

Circuit 1   Perform Exercises 1 to 2   Repeat 3x Total   No Rest

Sit Ups w twist   Set 1: 25   Set 2: 25-50   Set 3: 25-50

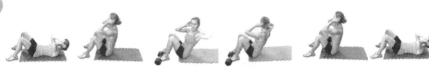

Leg Flutters   Set 1: 1 min   Set 2: 30 sec - 1 min   Set 3: 30 sec - 1 min

 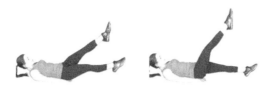

Circuit 2   Perform Exercises 1 to 4, Repeat 4x No Rest

Stand Ups (each leg)   Set 1: 20   Set 2: 20   Set 3: 20   Set 4: 20

Star Jumps   Set 1: 25   Set 2: 50   Set 3: 50   Set 4: 50

  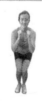

One Arm Row   Set 1: 15   Set 2: 12   Set 3: 12   Set 4: 8

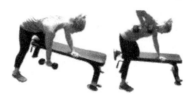

High Plank Rowing (each arm)   Set 1: 5   Set 2: 5-10   Set 3: 5-10   Set 4: 5-10

 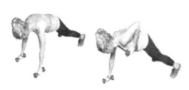

Body Reboot Transformations

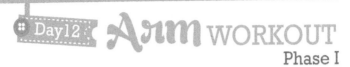

Day 12 — **Arm** WORKOUT

Phase I

Jog or Power Walk 3-5 miles

Body Reboot Transformations

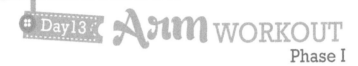

Day 13 — **Arm** WORKOUT

Phase I

Circuit 1   Perform exercises 1 to 5, Repeat 4x No Rest

Jump Rope or Jumping Jacks with a Fist   Set 1: 1 min   Set 2: 2 min   Set 3: 2 min   Set 4: 2 min

①

Standing Curls   Set 1: 25   Set 2: 15   Set 3: 10   Set 4: 10

②

45 Degree Chest Press   Set 1: 12   Set 2: 12   Set 3: 12   Set 4: 8

③

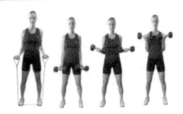

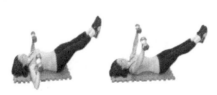

Regular Push Ups   Set 1: 15-20   Set 2: 25-30   Set 3: 25-50   Set 4: 15-20

 4

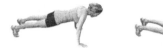 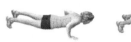

Mountain Climbers   Set 1: 1 min   Set 2: 1 min   Set 4:1 min

5

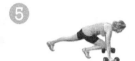 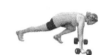

Circuit 2   Perform exercises 1 to 4, Repeat 3x No Rest

Squats   Set 1: 50   Set 2: 50   Set 3: 50

 1

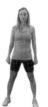 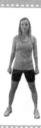

Hammer Curls   Set 1: 25   Set 2: 25   Set 3: 25

2

  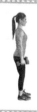

Concentration Curls   Set 1: 15   Set 2: 12   Set 3: 8-12

 3

Push Ups Pulses   Set 1: 25   Set 2: 25   Set 3: 25

 4

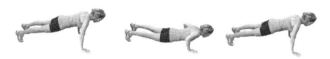

Circuit 3

Perform Exercises 1 to 4, Repeat 3x No Rest

Hip Raises   Set 1: 50   Set 2: 50-100   Set 3: 50-100

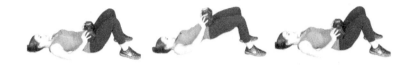

Good Mornings   Set 1: 12   Set 2: 12   Set 3: 12

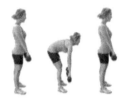

Back leg Curls (ball)   Set 1: 20   Set 2: 20-30   Set 3: 20-30

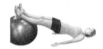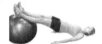

Alternate Lunge (each side)   Set 1: 10   Set 2: 10   Set 3: 10

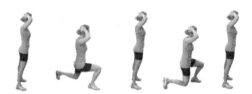
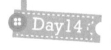

Body Reboot Transformations

Day 14   ARMWORKOUT
Phase I

Cardio 45-90 minutes

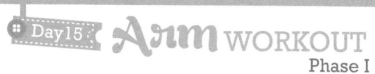

Body Reboot Transformations

Day 15 : Arm WORKOUT
Phase I

Circuit 1
Perform Exercises 1 to 5, Repeat 3x No Rest

Jump Rope or Jumping Jacks   set 1: 1 min   set 2: 2 min   set 3: 3 min

Regular Push Ups (knees)   Set 1: 10   Set 2: 10   Set 3: 10

 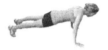 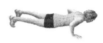 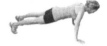

Triangle Push Ups (knees)   Set 1: 10   Set 2: 10   Set 3: 10

  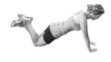 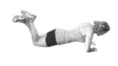

Tricep Push Backs   Set 1: 20   Set 2: 20   Set 3: 20

 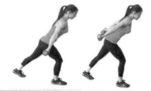

Jumping Squats   Set 1: 25   Set 2: 30   Set 3: 30

Circuit 2

Perform Exercises 1 to 4, Repeat 3x No Rest

Run High Knee   Set 1: 1 min   Set 2: 1 min   Set 3: 1 min

Punch Up High (with 2-3lbs dbs)   Set 1: 30 sec   Set 2: 30 sec   Set 3: 1 min

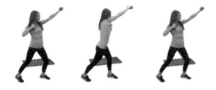

Burpees w dumbbells   Set 1: 15   Set 2: 15   Set 3: 15

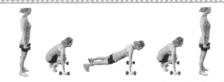

Star Jumps   Set 1: 25   Set 2: 50   Set 3: 50

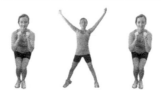

Circuit 3

Perform Exercises 1 to 5, Repeat 3x No Rest

Skating   Set 1: 1 min   Set 2: 2 min   Set 3: 2 min

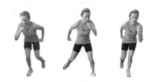

Low To High Plank (each Arm)   Set 1: 15-20   Set 2: 15-20   Set 3: 15-20

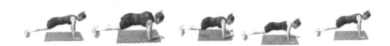

Mountain Climbers   Set 1: 1 min   Set 2: 1 min   Set 3: 1 min

③

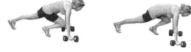

Plank with Walking   Set 1: 1 min   Set 2: 1 min   Set 3: 1 min

④

Back N Forth Hold Medicine Ball   Set 1: 30 sec   Set 2: 30 sec   Set 3: 30 sec

⑤

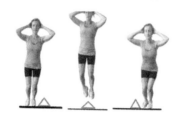

Body Reboot Transformations

Day 16 Arm WORKOUT
Phase I

• Jog or Power Walk 2-3 miles

Circuit 1   Perform Exercises 1 to 6, Repeat 3x No Rest

Sit Ups   Set 1: 1 min   Set 2: 1 min   Set 3: 1 min

①

Knee Tucks   Set 1: 25   Set 2: 50   Set 3: 50

②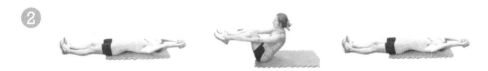

Bicycle   Set 1: 30 sec   Set 2: 1 min   Set 3: 1 min

③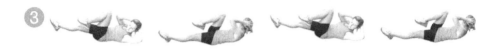

Plank   Set 1: 1 min   Set 2: 1 min   Set 3: 1-2 min

④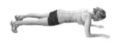

Leg Raises   Set 1: 15-25   Set 2: 15-25   Set 3: 15-25

⑤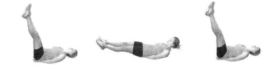

Plank On Ball   Set 1: 1 min   Set 2: 1 min   Set 3: 1 min

⑥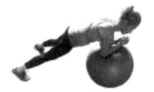

Circuit 2   Perform Exercises 1 to 5, Repeat 4x No Rest

Shoulder Press (Dumbbells)   Set 1: 12   Set 2: 12   Set 3: 8   Set 4: 8

①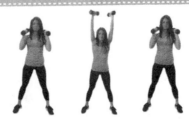

Side Raises (Dumbbells)   Set 1: 10   Set 2: 10   Set 3: 10   Set 4: 8

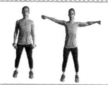

Bent Over Raises (Dumbbells)   Set 1: 15   Set 2: 15   Set 3: 12   Set 4: 12

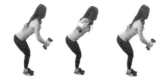

Kettle Bell Swing (db or kb)   Set 1: 30 sec   Set 2: 1 min   Set 3: 1 min   Set 4: 1 min

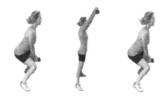

Jump Rope Or High Knee Running   Set 1: 1 min   Set 2: 1 min   Set 3: 2 min   Set 4: 2 min

Body Reboot Transformations

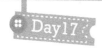 Day 17 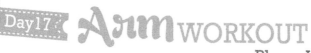 Arm WORKOUT

Phase I

- Jog 1 mile

Stretch 5 to 10 minutes (hamstring, quads, calves, lower and upper back)
Sprints @ 80% max (not full sprint), 3 x 25 yards or 3 x 15 sec on treadmill
Sprints @ 80% max, 5 x 50 yards or 5 x 30 sec on treadmill
Sprints@ 100 % max, 3 x 100 yards or 3 x 1 minute on treadmill

*rest 30 sec to 1 minute between sprints depending on fitness level. If you are a
beginner simply trot at 50-60% max. Don't sprint!

Circuit 1   Perform Exercises 1 to 4, Repeat 3 No Rest

Jump Rope or Jumping Jacks with a Fist   Set 1: 1 min   Set 2: 2 min   Set 3: 2 min

High Knee Running   Set 1: 1 min   Set 2: 1 min Set 3: 1 min

Back N Forth   Set 1: 1 min   Set 2: 1 min   Set 3: 1 min

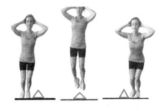

Skating   Set 1: 1 min   Set 2: 2 min   Set 3: 2 min

Circuit 2   Perform Exercises 1 to 8, Repeat 3x No Rest

Standing Curls (dumbbells)   Set 1: 10   Set 2: 10   Set 3: 10

 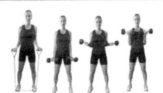

Standing Curls (dumbbells, heavier)   Set 1: 5-10   Set 2: 5-10   Set 3: 5-10

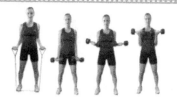

i.e. First exercise standing curls with 10 lbs Second exercise standing curls 15-20 lbs.

Hammer Curls (dumbbells)   Set 1: 10   Set 2: 20   Set 3: 30

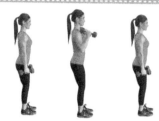

Overhead Tricep Extensions   Set 1: 20   Set 2: 20   Set 3: 20

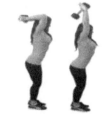

Tricep Push Backs   Set 1: 15   Set 2: 15-20   Set 3: 15-20

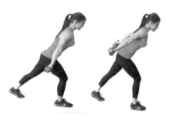

*Tricep Bench Dips w db on Legs   Set 1: 20   Set 2: 30   Set 3: 30

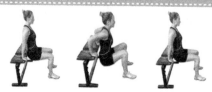

*place a dumbbell on your thighs horizontal, 15-30lb. Feet 3-4 inches apart, bent knee, keep back sliding along edge of bench with every rep, squeeze tricep on top.

Concentration Curls (each arm) Set 1: 20   Set 2: 10   Set 3: 10

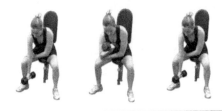

Regular Push Ups Set 1: 10-20   Set 2: 10-20   Set 3: 10-20

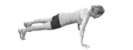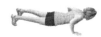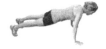

Cardio

Jog 1 mile

Sprints @80-90% Jog 50 yards, turn and sprint 50 yards. Repeat 3x no rest if possible. Rest 1 minute and Repeat 1x.

Body Reboot Transformations

Day 18 Arm WORKOUT
Phase I

Cardio 30 minutes

Circuit 1 Perform Exercises 1 to 3, Repeat 3x NoRest

Sit Ups w twist Set 1: 25-50   Set 2: 25-50   Set 3: 25-50

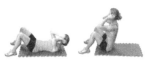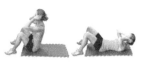

Leg Flutters Set 1: 1 min   Set 2: 30 sec - 1 min   Set 3: 30 sec - 1 min

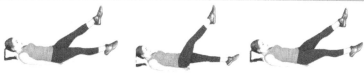

Leg Raises (90 deg to 3") Set 1: 25   Set 2: 25   Set 3: 25-50

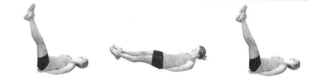

Circuit 2   Perform Exercises 1 to 6, Repeat 4 No Rest

Squats w Dumbbell Set 1: 15   Set 2: 15   Set 3: 15   Set 4: 15

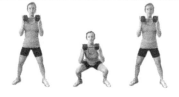

Stand Ups (each leg) Set 1: 20   Set 2: 20   Set 3: 20   Set 4: 20

Star Jumps Set 1: 25   Set 2: 50   Set 3: 50   Set 4: 50

One arm Row Set 1: 15   Set 2: 12   Set 3: 12   Set 4: 8

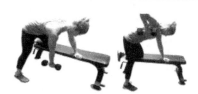

High Plank Rowing (each arm)   Set 1: 5   Set 2: 5-10   Set 3: 5-10   Set 4: 5-10

⑤

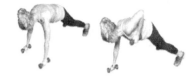

Bent Over Rows   Set 1:10   Set 2: 10   Set 3: 8-12   Set 4: 8-12

⑥

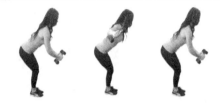

Body Reboot Transformations

 Day19 **Arm** WORKOUT
Phase I

Cardio

- Jog or Power Walk 3-6 miles

Body Reboot Transformations

 Day20 WORKOUT
Phase I

Circuit 1   Perform Exercises 1 to 6, Repeat 4x

Jump Rope or Jumping Jacks with a Fist   Set 1: 1 min   Set 2: 2 min   Set 3: 2 min   Set 4: 2 min

①

Hammer Curls   Set 1: 25   Set 2: 15   Set 3: 10   Set 4: 10

 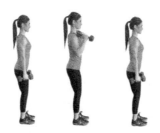

45 Degree Chest Press   Set 1: 12   Set 2: 12   Set 3: 12   Set 4: 8

 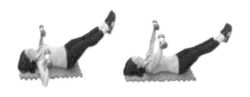

Regular Push Ups   Set 1: 15-20   Set 2: 25-30   Set 3: 25-50   Set 4: 15-20

 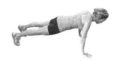 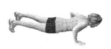 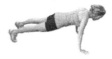

Push ups w/ knees on box or ball   Set 1: 10   Set 2: 10-15   Set 3: 10-15   Set 4: 10-15

 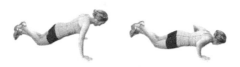

Mountain Climbers   Set 1: 1 min   Set 2: 1 min   Set 3: 1 min   Set 4: 1 min

Circuit 2

Perform Exercises 1 to 5, Repeat 3x No Rest

Squats   Set 1: 50   Set 2: 50   Set 3: 50

 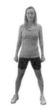 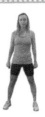

Walking Lunge   Set 1: 2 min   Set 2: 2 min   Set 3: 2 min

Hammer Curls   Set 1: 25   Set 2: 25   Set 3: 25

 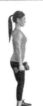 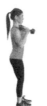 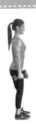

Concentration Curls   Set 1: 15   Set 2: 12   Set 3: 8-12

   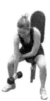

Push Ups Pulses   Set 1: 25   Set 2: 25-50   Set 3: 25-50

 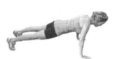 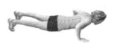 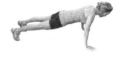

Circuit 3

Perform Exercises 1 to 4, Repeat 3x No Rest

Hip Raises   Set 1: 50   Set 2: 50-100   Set 3: 50-100

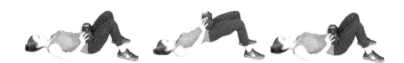

One leg Hip Raises (each leg)   Set 1: 25   Set 2: 25-50   Set 3: 25-50

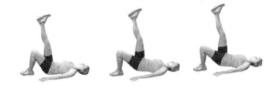

Good Mornings   Set 1: 12   Set 2: 12   Set 3: 12

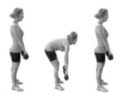

Back leg Curls (ball)   Set 1: 20   Set 2: 20-30   Set 3: 20-30

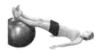

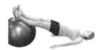

Body Reboot Transformations

Day 21 Arm WORKOUT
Phase I

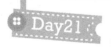

Cardio 45-90 minutes

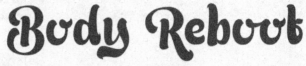

Body Reboot

transformation series

Lean Great Arms & Abs

Phase II

Body Reboot Transformations

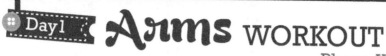

Day 1 · Arms WORKOUT
Phase II

Circuit 1
Perform Exercises 1 to 3, Repeat 3x, No Rest

Jump Rope or Jumping Jacks set 1: 1 min set 2: 2 min set 3: 3 min

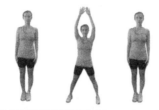

Regular Push Ups (knees) Set 1: 10 Set 2: 15 Set 3: 20

Jumping Squats Set 1: 25 Set 2: 30 Set 3: 30

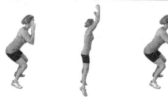

Circuit 2
Perform Exercises 1 to 4, Repeat 3x Total, No Rest

Run High Knee Set 1: 1 min Set 2: 1 min Set 3: 1 min

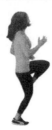

Punch Up High (with 2-3lbs dbs) Set 1: 30 sec   Set 2: 30 sec   Set 3: 30 sec

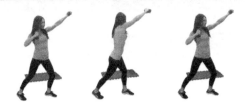

Burpees Set 1: 10   Set 2: 30   Set 3: 30

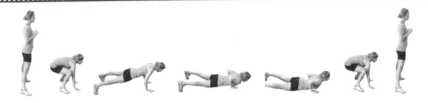

Kettle Bell or Db Swing (15lb) Set 1: 1 min   Set 2: 1 min   Set 3: 1 min

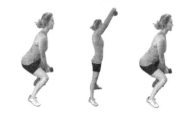

Circuit 3

Skating Set 1: 1 min   Set 2: 1 min   Set 3: 1 min

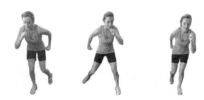

Low To High Plank (each Arm) Set 1: 15-20   Set 2: 15-20   Set 3: 15

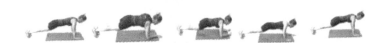

Kick backs (each arm)   Set 1: 10   Set 2: 10   Set 3: 10

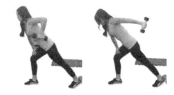

Mountain Climbers   Set 1: 1 min   Set 2: 1 min   Set 3: 1 min

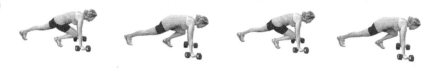

High Plank   Set 1: 1 min   Set 2: 1 min   Set 3: 1 min

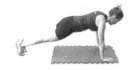

Body Reboot Transformations

Day2   Arms WORKOUT
Phase II

Cardio

- Jog or Power Walk   2-4 miles

Circuit 1   Perform Each Exercises 1 to 4   Repeat 3x   No Rest

Sit Ups   Set 1: 1 min   Set 2: 1 min   Set 3: 1 min

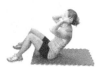

Knee Tucks Set 1: 25 Set 2: 50 Set 3: 50

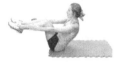

Bicycle Set 1 : 1 min Set 2 : 1 min Set 3 : 1 min

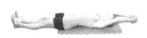

Plank Set 1: 1 min Set 2: 1 min Set 3: 1 min

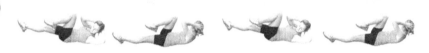

Circuit 2 Perform Exercises 1 to 5, Repeat 4x, No Rest

Shoulder Press (Dumbbells) Set 1: 12 Set 2: 12 Set 3: 12

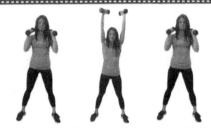

Light, i.e. 5-8lbs

Side Raises (Dumbbells) Set 1: 10 Set 2: 10 Set 3: 10 Set 4: 8

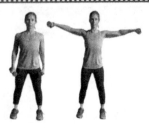

High Plank Rowing (each arm) Set 1: 5 Set 2: 5 Set 3: 5 Set 4: 5

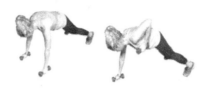

Bent Over Raises (Dumbbells) Set 1: 12 Set 2: 12 Set 3: 12 Set 4: 12

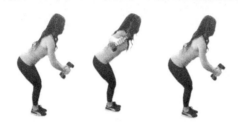

Squat and Press (Dumbbells) Set 1: 8 Set 2: 8 Set 3: 8 Set 4: 8

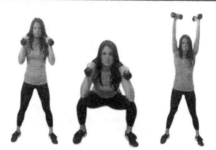

Heavy, i.e. 10-20lbs.

Body Reboot Transformations

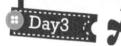 Day3 Arm WORKOUT
Phase II

Jog 1 mile

Stretch 5 to 10 minutes (hamstring, quads, calves, lower and upper back)
Sprints @ 80% max (not full sprint), 3 x 25 yards or 3 x 15 sec on treadmill
Sprints @ 90% max, 6 x 50 yards or 6 x 30 sec on treadmill

*Rest 30 sec to 1 minute between sprints depending on fitness level. If you are a beginner simply trot at50% max. Don't sprint!

Circuit 1   Perform Exercises 1 to 5, Repeat 3x Total, No Rest

Jump Rope or Jumping Jacks with a Fist   Set 1: 1 min   Set 2: 2 min   Set 3: 2 min

 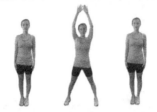

High Knee Running   Set 1: 1 min   Set 2: 1 min   Set 3: 1 min

Mountain Climbers   Set 1: 1 min   Set 2: 1 min   Set 3: 1 min

 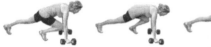 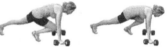

Burpees   Set 1: 10   Set 2: 20   Set 3: 20

 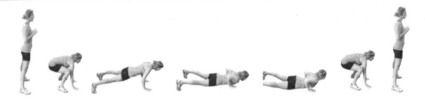

Back N Forth   Set 1: 1 min   Set 2: 1 min   Set 3: 1 min

Circuit 2 Perform Exercise 1 to 3 Repeat 3x Total No Rest

Standing Curls (dumbbells) Set 1: 10 Set 2: 20 Set 3: 20

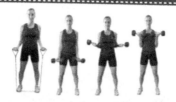

Standing Curls (blue or red band) Set 1: 30 sec Set 2: 30 sec Set 3: 30 sec

Skating Set 1: 1 min Set 2: 1 min set 3: 1 min

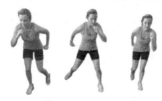

Hammer Curls (dumbbell) Set 1: 10 Set 2: 20 Set 3: 30

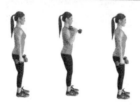

Overhead Tricep Extensions Set 1: 20 Set 2: 20 Set 3: 20

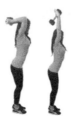

Tricep Push Ups (knees)   Set 1: 10-20   Set 2: 10-20   Set 3: 10-20

4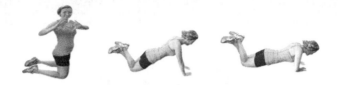

Tricep Bench Dips   Set 1: 30   Set 2: 30   Set 3: 30

5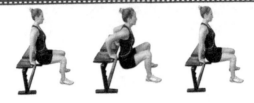

Cardio

Jog 1 mile

Body Reboot Transformations

Day 4   **Arm** WORKOUT
Phase II

Cardio 30 minutes

Circuit 1   Perform Exercise 1 to 3   Repeat 3x Total   No Rest

Knee Tucks   Set 1: 25   Set 2: 50   Set 3: 50

1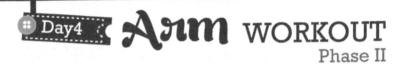

Cross Over (each side)   Set 1: 25   Set 2: 25   Set 3: 25

2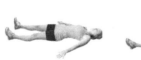

Sit Ups w twist   Set 1: 25   Set 2: 50   Set 3: 50

3

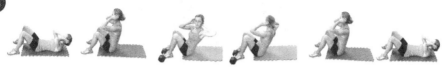

Leg Raises 90 to 3"   Set 1: 25   Set 2: 25   Set 3: 25

4

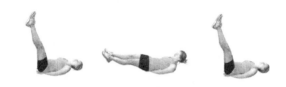

Bicycle   Set 1: 1 min   Set 2: 1 min   Set 3: 1 min

5

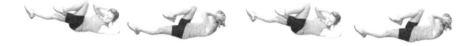

Circuit 2   Perform Exercise 1 to 5, Repeat 4x Total, No Rest

Stand Ups (each leg)   Set 1: 25   Set 2: 25   Set 3: 25   Set 4: 25

1

Star Jumps   Set 1: 50   Set 2: 50   Set 3: 50   Set 4: 25

2

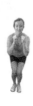
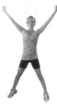

One arm Row   Set 1: 15   Set 2: 12   Set 3: 8   Set 4: 8

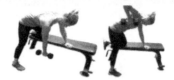

Kettle Bell or Db Swing   Set 1: 1 min   Set 2: 1 min   Set 3: 1 min   Set 4: 1 min

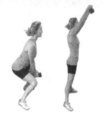

Burpees w/ dumbbell   Set 1: 15   Set 2: 15   set 3: 15   Set 4: 15

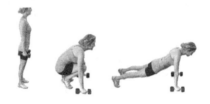

Burpees   Set 1: 25   Set 2: 25   set 3: 25   Set 4: 25

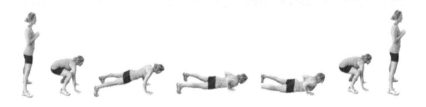

Body Reboot Transformations

Day5   **Arm** WORKOUT
Phase II

Jog or Power Walk 3-6 miles

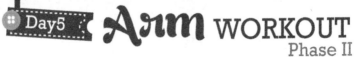

Body Reboot Transformations

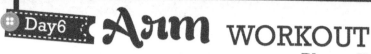

Day 6 · *Arm* WORKOUT

Phase II

Circuit 1   Perform Exercise 1 to 5, Repeat 4x, No Rest

10 Jumping Jacks, 5 push ups   Set 1: 1 min   Set 2: 2 min   Set 3: 2 min   Set 4: 2 min

①

Standing Curls   Set 1: 25   Set 2: 15   Set 3: 10   Set 4: 10

②

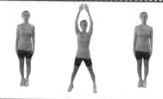

45 Degree Chest Press   Set 1: 12   Set 2: 12   Set 3: 12   Set 4: 8

③

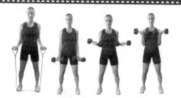

Regular Push Ups   Set 1: 15-20   Set 2: 25-30   Set 3: 25-50   Set 4: 15-20

④

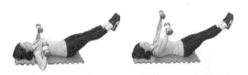

Tricep Push Backs.   Set 1: 1 min   Set 2: 1 min   Set 3: 1 min   Set 4: 30 sec

⑤

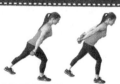

Circuit 2   <small>Perform Exercise 1 to 5, Repeat 3x, No Rest</small>

Mountain Climbers   <small>Set 1: 2 min   Set 2: 2 min   Set 3: 1 min</small>

   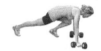

Hammer Curls   <small>Set 1: 25   Set 2: 25   Set 3: 25</small>

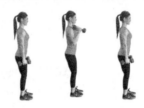

Concentration Curls   <small>Set 1: 15   Set 2: 12   Set 3: 8-12</small>

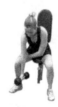 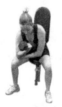 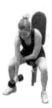

Tricep Bench w db   <small>Set 1: 20   Set 2: 20   Set 3: 20</small>

Push Ups Pulses   <small>Set 1: 25   Set 2: 25   Set 3: 25</small>

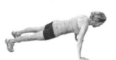 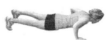 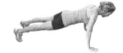

Circuit 3

Perform Exercises 1 to 5, Repeat 3x No Rest

Hip Raises   Set 1: 50   Set 2: 50-100   Set 3: 50-100

1

Good Mornings   Set 1: 12   Set 2: 12   Set 3: 12

2

Back Leg Curls (ball)   Set 1: 20   Set 2: 20-30   Set 3: 20-30

3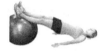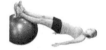

Jumping Squat w* wght   Set 1: 20   Set 2: 20   Set 3: 20

4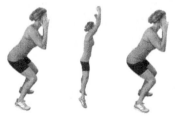

High Plank Rowing (each side)   Set 1: 5-8   Set 2: 5-8   Set 3: 5-8

5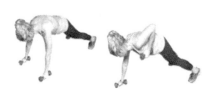

Body Reboot Transformations

⬢ Day7 ⎯ Arm WORKOUT
Phase II

Cardio 60-90 minutes

Body Reboot Transformations

⬢ Day8 ⎯ Arm WORKOUT
Phase II

Circuit 1   **Perform Exercises 1 to 5, Repeat 3x No Rest**

Jump Rope or Jumping Jacks   set 1: 1 min   set 2: 2 min   set 3: 3 min

1

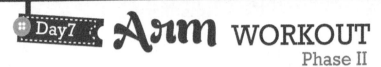

Regular Push Ups   Set 1: 10   Set 2: 20   Set 3: 20

2

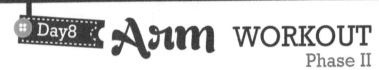

Triangle Push Ups (knees)   Set 1: 20   Set 2: 20   Set 3: 20

3

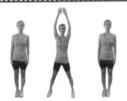

Tricep Kick Backs (light 3-5lbs)   Set 1: 20   Set 2: 20   Set 3:20

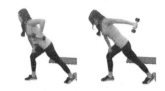

Mt Climbers   Set 1: 1 min   Set 2: 1 min   Set 3: 1 min

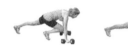

Circuit 2   Perform Exercises 1 to 5, Repeat 3x No Rest

Run High Knee   Set 1: 1 min   Set 2: 1 min   Set 3: 1 min

Punch Up High (with 2-3lbs dbs)   Set 1: 30 sec   Set 2: 30 sec   et 3: 30 sec

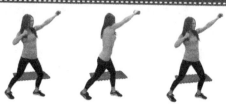

Burpees w a star jump   Set 1: 25   Set 2: 25   Set 3: 25

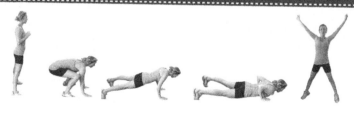

Back N Forth · Set 1: 1 min Set 2: 2 min Set 3; 2 min

 ④

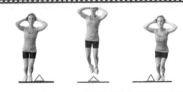

Skating · Set 1: 1 min Set 2: 1 min Set 3: 1 min

⑤

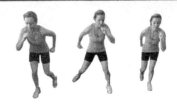

Circuit 3 · Perform Exercise 1 to 5, Repeat 3x No Rest

Jump Rope · Set 1: 1 min Set 2: 2 min Set 3: 2 min

①

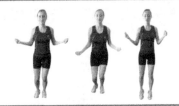

Low To High Plank (each Arm) · Set 1: 20-25 Set 2: 15-25 Set 3: 15-25

②

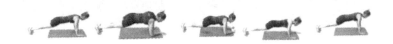

Sprint (start to 50 yards or 30 sec treadmill)

③

Set 1: repeat 6x   Set 2: repeat 5x   Set 3: Repeat 4x

Plank with walking · Set 1: 1 min Set 2: 1 min Set 3: 1 min

④

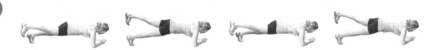

Tricep Push Backs
Set 1: 30   Set 2: 20   Set 3: 10 (heavy i.e. 15-20lbs)

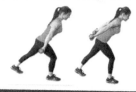

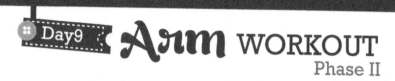

Body Reboot Transformations
Day9   Arm WORKOUT
Phase II

Jog or Power Walk 2-3 miles

Circuit 1
Perform Exercise 1 to 6, Repeat 3x No rest

Sit Ups   Set 1: 1 min   Set 2: 1 min   Set 3: 1 min

Knee Tucks   Set 1: 25   Set 2: 50   Set 3: 50

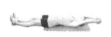

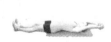

Bicycle   Set 1: 30 sec   Set 2: 1 min   Set 3: 1 min

Plank   Set 1: 1 min   Set 2: 1 min Set 3: 1-2 min

Leg Raises   Set 1: 15-25   Set 2: 15-25   Set 3: 15-25

5

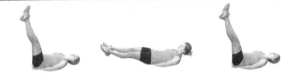

Kickouts   Set 1: 20   Set 2: 20   Set 3: 20

6

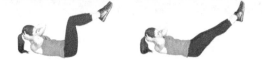

Circuit 2   Perform Exercises 1 to 5, Repeat 4x No Rest

Shoulder Press (Dumbbells)   Set 1: 12   Set 2: 12   Set 3: 8   Set 4: 8

1

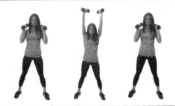

Side Raises (Dumbbells)   Set 1: 10   Set 2: 10   Set 3: 10   Set 4: 8

2

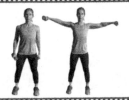

One Arm Row (each arm)   Set 1: 15   Set 2: 12   Set 3: 10   Set 4: 10

2

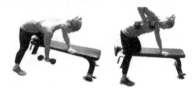

Bent Over Raises (Dumbbells)   Set 1: 15   Set 2: 15   Set 3: 12   Set 4: 12

3

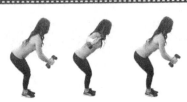

Body Reboot Transformations

Day 10 — Arm WORKOUT
Phase II

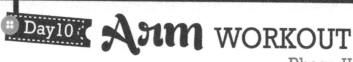

Jog 1 mile

Stretch 5 to 10 minutes (hamstring, quads, calves, lower and upper back)
Sprints @ 80% max (not full sprint), 3 x 25 yards or 3 x 15 sec on treadmill
Sprints @ 80% max, 5 x 50 yards or 5 x 30 sec on treadmill
Sprints@ 100 % max, 2 x 100 yards or 2 x 1 minute on treadmill
*rest 30 sec to 1 minute between sprints depending on fitness level. If you are a beginner
simply trot at 50% max. Don't sprint!

Circuit 1   Perform Exercises 1 to 3, Repeat 3x No Rest

Jump Rope or Jumping Jacks with a Fist   Set 1: 2 min   Set 2: 2 min   Set 3: 2 min

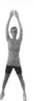

Back N Forth   Set 1: 1 min   Set 2: 1 min   Set 3: 1 min

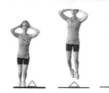

Skating   Set 1: 1 min   Set 2: 1 min   Set 3: 1 min

❸

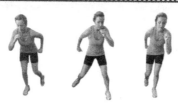

Circuit 2   <small>Perform Exercises 1 to 6, Repeat 3x No rest</small>

Standing Curls (dumbbells)   Set 1: 10 Set 2: 10 Set 3: 10

 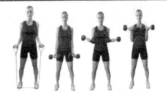

Concentration curls (dumbbells, heavier)   Set 1: 5-10 Set 2: 5-10 Set 3: 5-10

 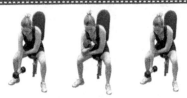

Hammer Curls (dumbbells)   Set 1: 10 Set 2: 20 Set 3: 30

 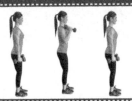

Overhead Tricep Extensions   Set 1: 20 Set 2: 20 Set 3: 20reps

Tricep Push Backs   Set 1: 15 Set 2: 15 Set 3: 8 (heavy)

 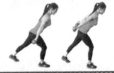

Tricep Bench Dips w db   Set 1: 30 Set 2: 30 Set 3: 30

 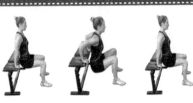

Cardio

Jog 1- 3 Mile

Body Reboot Transformations

Day 11 — **Arm** WORKOUT

Phase II

Cardio 30 minutes

Circuit 1 Perform Exercises 1 to 4   Repeat 3x Total   No Rest

Sit Ups w twist   Set 1: 25   Set 2: 25-50   Set 3: 25-50

1

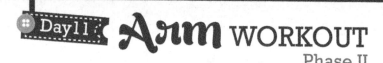

Knee Tucks   Set 1: 50   Set 2: 50   Set 3: 50

2

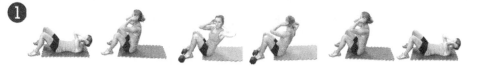

Bicycle   Set 1: 1 min   Set 2: 1 min   Set 3: 1 min

3

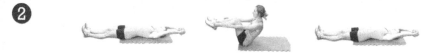

Circuit 2 Perform Exercises 1 to 5, Repeat 4x No Rest

Stand Ups (each leg)   Set 1: 20   Set 2: 20   Set 3: 20   Set 4: 20

1

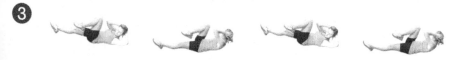

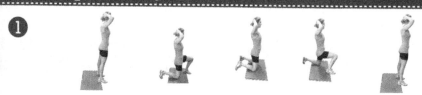

Star Jumps   Set 1: 25   Set 2: 50   Set 3: 50   Set 4: 50

One Arm Row   Set 1: 15   Set 2: 12   Set 3: 12   Set 4: 8

 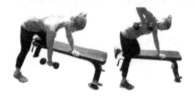

High Plank Rowing (each arm)   Set 1: 5   Set 2: 5-10   Set 3: 5-10   Set 4: 5-10

 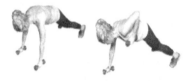

Kettle Bell or Db Swing   Set 1: 1 min   Set 2: 1 min   Set 3: 1 min   Set 4: 1 min

 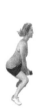 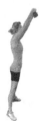 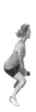

Body Reboot Transformations

 Day 12   # Arm WORKOUT
Phase II

Jog or Power Walk 3-7 miles

Body Reboot Transformations

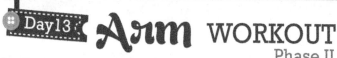

Day 13 *Arm* WORKOUT
Phase II

Circuit 1 Perform Exercise 1 to 7, Repeat 4x No Rest

Jump Rope or Jumping Jacks with a Fist   Set 1: 1 min   Set 2: 2 min   Set 3: 2 min   Set 4: 2 min

1

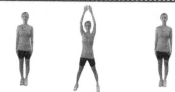

Standing Curls   Set 1: 25   Set 2: 15   Set 3: 10   Set 4: 10

2

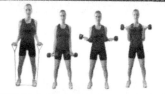

45 Degree Chest Press   Set 1: 12   Set 2: 12   Set 3: 12   Set 4: 8

3

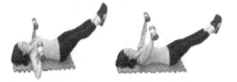

Flies with fitness Ball   Set 1: 15   Set 2: 15   Set 3: 15   Set 4: 15

4

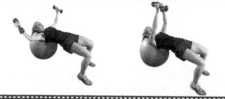

Burpees   Set 1: 10   Set 2: 10   Set 3: 10   Set 4: 10

5

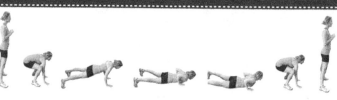

Regular Push Ups   Set 1: 15-20   Set 2: 25-30   Set 3: 25-50   Set 4: 25-50

⑥
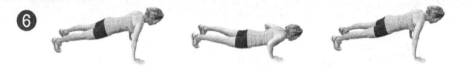

Mountain Climbers   Set 1: 1 min   Set 2: 1 min   Set 3: 1 min   Set 4: 2 min

⑦
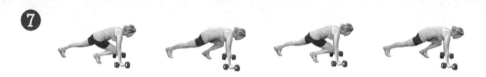

Circuit 2   Perform Exercise 1 to 6, Repeat 3x No Rest

Squats   Set 1: 50   Set 2: 50   Set 3: 50

①
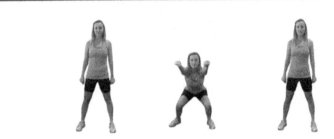

Hip Raises with weight   Set 1: 25   Set 2: 25   Set 3: 25-50

②
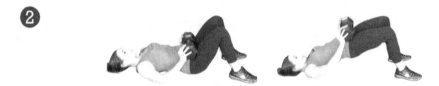

Hammer Curls   Set 1: 25   Set 2: 25   Set 3: 25

③
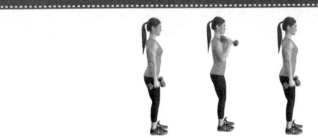

Concentration Curls (each arm)   Set 1: 15   Set 2: 12   Set 3: 8-12

 4

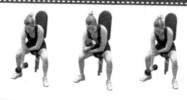

Push Ups Pulses   Set 1: 25   Set 2: 25   Set 3: 25

 5

Tricep Push Backs   Set 1: 20   Set 2: 15   Set 3: 10

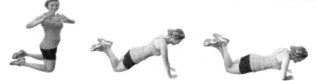 **6**

Circuit 3   Perform Exercise 1 to 5, Repeat 3x   No Rest

Hip Raises (with weight)   Set 1: 50   Set 2: 50-100   Set 3: 50-100

 1

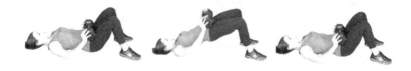

Good Mornings   Set 1: 12   Set 2: 12   Set 3: 12

2

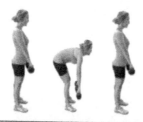

Back Leg Curls (ball)   Set 1: 20   Set 2: 20-30   Set 3: 20-30

3

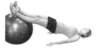 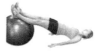

Lunge 3 to 4 (each side)   Set 1: 10   Set 2 : 10   Set 3: 10

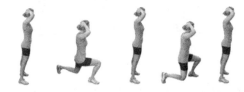

Split Squat   Set 1: 30 sec   Set 2: 30 sec   Set 3: 30 sec

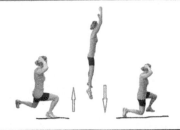

Body Reboot Transformations

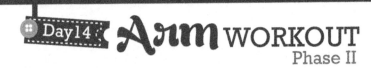

:: Day 14 ⟩ Arm WORKOUT
Phase II

Cardio 60-90 minutes

Body Reboot Transformations

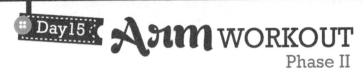

:: Day 15 ⟩ Arm WORKOUT
Phase II

Circuit 1   Perform Exercises 1 to 5, Repeat 3x No Rest

10 Jumping Jacks, 5 push ups   set 1: 1 min   set 2: 2 min   set 3: 3 min

Shoulder Press Set 1: 20 Set 2: 20 Set 3: 30 (light)

2

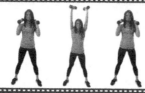

Triangle Push Ups (knees) Set 1: 10 Set 2: 10 Set 3: 10

3

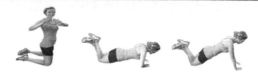

Tricep Push Backs Set 1: 20 Set 2: 20 Set 3: 20

4

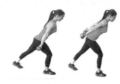

Jumping Squats Set 1: 25 Set 2: 30 Set 3: 30

5

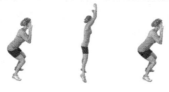

Circuit 2 Perform Exercise 1 to 4, Repeat 3x No Rest

Run High Knee Set 1: 1 min Set 2: 1 min Set 3: 1 min

1

Punch Up High (with 2-3lbs dbs) Set 1: 30 sec Set 2: 1 min Set 3: 1 min

2

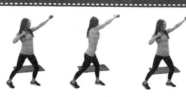

Burpees w dumbbells Set 1: 15   Set 2: 25   Set 3: 25

 ③

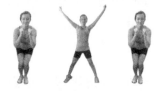

Star Jumps Set 1: 25   Set 2: 50   Set 3: 50

④

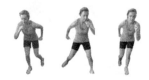

Circuit 3 Perform Exercise 1 to 6, Repeat 3x No Rest

Skating Set 1: 1 min   Set 2: 2 min   Set 3: 2 min

①

Low To High Plank (each Arm) Set 1: 15-20   Set 2: 15-20   Set 3: 15-20

②

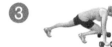   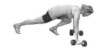

Mountain Climbers Set 1: 2 min   Set 2: 2 min   Set 3: 2 min

③

High Plank Rowing Set 1: 1 min   Set 2: 1 min   Set 3: 1 min

④

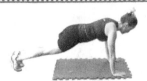

Back N Forth Hold mb   Set 1: 2 min   Set 2: 2 min   Set 3: 2 min

⑤

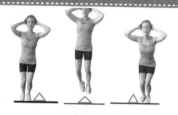

One Arm Row   Set 1: 15   Set 2: 8 (heavy)   Set 3: 6 (heavier)

⑥

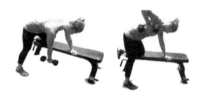

Body Reboot Transformations

Day 16 Arm WORKOUT

Phase II

• Jog or Power Walk 2-3 miles

Circuit 1   Perform Exercise 1 to 6, Repeat 3x No Rest

Sit Ups   Set 1: 1 min   Set 2: 1 min   Set 3: 1 min

❶

  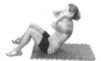

Knee Tucks   Set 1: 25   Set 2: 50   Set 3: 50

❷

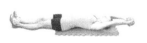 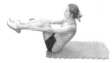 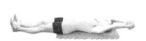

Bicycle Set 1: 1 min   Set 2: 1 min   Set 3: 1 min

3

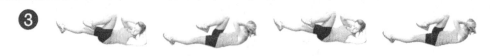

Plank Set 1: 1 min   Set 2: 1 min   Set 3: 1-2 min

4

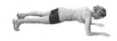

Leg Raises Set 1: 15-25   Set 2: 15-25   Set 3: 15-25

5

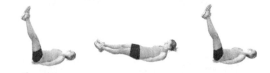

Plank On Ball Set 1: 2 min   Set 2: 2 min   Set 3: 2 min

6

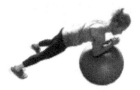

Circuit 2 Perform Exercise 1 to 7, Repeat 4x No Rest

Shoulder Press (Dumbbells) Set 1: 12   Set 2: 12   Set 3: 8   Set 4: 8

1

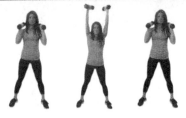

Side Raises (Dumbbells) Set 1: 10   Set 2: 10   Set 3: 10   Set 4: 8

2

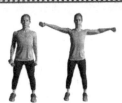

Bent Over Raises (Dumbbells)   Set 1: 15   Set 2: 15   Set 3: 12   Set 4: 12

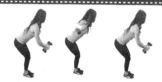

Kettle Bell Swing (db or kb)   Set 1: 30 sec   Set 2: 1 min   Set 3: 1 min   Set 4: 1 min

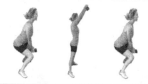

Jump Rope Or High Knee Running

Set 1: 1 min   Set 2: 1 min   Set 3: 2 min   Set 4: 2 min

Body Reboot Transformations

Day 17 Arm WORKOUT
Phase II

• Jog 2-3 Mile

Stretch 5 to 10 minutes (hamstring, quads, calves, lower and upper back)
Sprints @ 80% max (not full sprint), 3 x 25 yards or 3 x 15 sec on treadmill
Sprints @ 80% max, 5 x 50 yards or 5 x 30 sec on treadmill
Sprints@ 100 % max, 3 x 100 yards or 3 x 1 minute on treadmill

***rest 30 sec to 1 minute between sprints depending on fitness level. If you are a
beginner simply trot at 50-60% max. Don't sprint!**

Circuit 1   Perform Exercise 1 to 3, Repeat 4x No Rest

Standing Curls (dumbbells)   Set 1: 10   Set 2: 10   Set 3: 10   set 4: 10

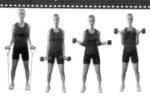

Standing Curls (dumbbells, heavier)   Set 1: 5-10   Set 2: 5-10   Set 3: 5-10   Set 4: 10

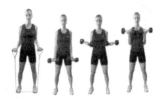

i.e. First exercise standing curls with 10 lbs Second exercise standing curls 15-20 lbs.

Hammer Curls (dumbbells)   Set 1: 10   Set 2: 20   Set 3: 30   Set 4: 30

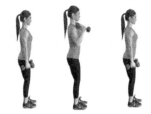

Circuit 2   Perform Exercise 1 to 7, Repeat 4x No Rest

Overhead Tricep Extensions   Set 1: 20   Set 2: 20   Set 3: 20   set 4: 20

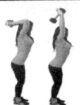

Tricep Push Ups   Set 1: 15   Set 2: 15-20   Set 3: 15-20   Set 4: 15-20

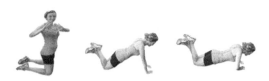

Cardio

Jog 1 mile

Sprints @80-90% Jog 50 yards, turn and sprint 50 yards. Repeat 3x no rest if possible. Rest 1 minute and Repeat 1x.

Body Reboot Transformations

Arm WORKOUT

Phase II

Cardio 30 minutes

Circuit 1   Perform Exercise 1 to 3, Repeat 3x No Rest

Sit Ups w twist   Set 1: 25-50   Set 2: 25-50   Set 3: 25-50

1

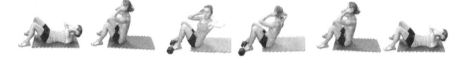

Leg Flutters   Set 1: 1 min   Set 2: 30 sec - 1 min   Set 3: 30 sec - 1 min

2

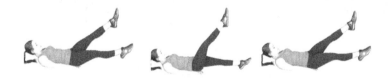

Leg Raises (90 deg to 3")   Set 1: 50   Set 2: 50   Set 3: 50

3

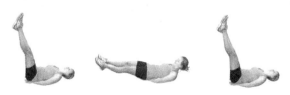

Circuit 2

Perform Exercise 1 to 6, Repeat 4x No Rest

Squats w Dumbbell   Set 1: 15   Set 2: 15   Set 3: 15   Set 4: 15

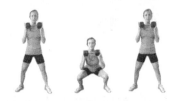

Stand Ups (each leg)   Set 1: 20   Set 2: 20   Set 3: 20   Set 4: 20

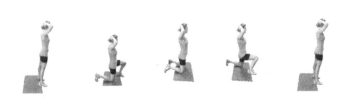

Star Jumps   Set 1: 25   Set 2: 50   Set 3: 50   Set 4: 50

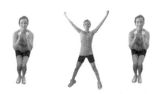

One arm Row   Set 1: 15   Set 2: 12   Set 3: 12   Set 4: 8

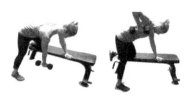

High Plank Rowing (each arm)   Set 1: 5   Set 2: 5-10   Set 3: 5-10   Set 4: 5-10

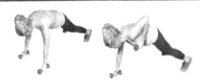

Bent Over Raises   Set 1:10   Set 2: 10   Set 3: 8-12   Set 4: 8-12

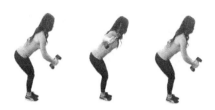

Body Reboot Transformations

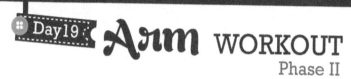

Day19 Arm WORKOUT
Phase II

Cardio

• Jog or Power Walk 4-6 miles

Body Reboot Transformations

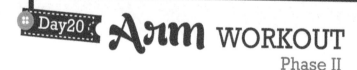

Day20 Arm WORKOUT
Phase II

Circuit 1   Perform Exercise 1 to 6, Repeat 4x No Rest

Jump Rope or Jumping Jacks with a Fist   Set 1: 1 min Set 2: 2 min Set 3: 2 min Set 4: 2 min

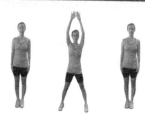

Regular Curls   Set 1: 25   Set 2: 15   Set 3: 10   Set 4: 10

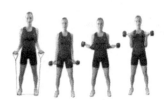

45 Degree Chest Press   Set 1: 12   Set 2: 12   Set 3: 12   Set 4: 8

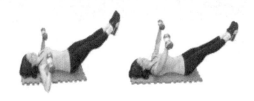

Regular Push Ups   Set 1: 15-20   Set 2: 25-30   Set 3: 25-50   Set 4: 15-20

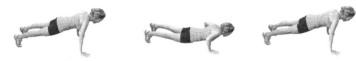
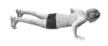
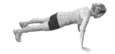

Push ups w/ knees on box or ball   Set 1: 10   Set 2: 10-15   Set 3: 10-15   Set 4: 10-15

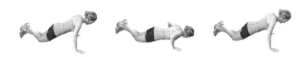

Mountain Climbers   Set 1: 1 min   Set 2: 1 min   Set 3: 1 min   Set 4: 1 min

Circuit 2   Perform Exercise 1 to 5, Repeat 3x No Rest

Squats   Set 1: 50   Set 2: 50   Set 3: 50

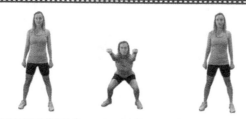

Lunge (each side)   Set 1: 10   Set 2: 10   Set 3: 15

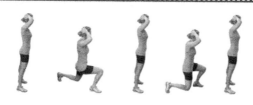

Hammer Curls   Set 1: 25   Set 2: 25   Set 3: 25

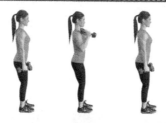

Concentration Curls   Set 1: 15   Set 2: 12   Set 3: 8-12

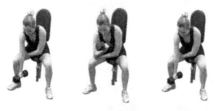

Push Ups Pulses   Set 1: 25   Set 2: 25-50   Set 3: 25-50

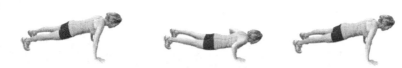

Circuit 3

Perform Exercise 1 to 4, Repeat 3x No Rest

Hip Raises (with weight)   Set 1: 50   Set 2: 50-100   Set 3: 50-100

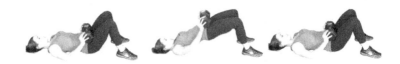

One Leg Hip Raises (each leg)   Set 1: 25   Set 2: 25-50   Set 3: 25-50

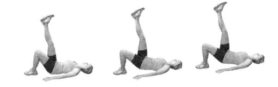

Good Mornings   Set 1: 12   Set 2: 12   Set 3: 12

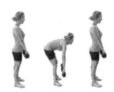

Back Leg Curls (ball)   Set 1: 20   Set 2: 20-30   Set 3: 20-30

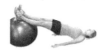

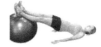

Body Reboot Transformations

Day21   Arm WORKOUT
Phase II

Cardio 60-90 minutes

21 DAY DIET

Mission: lose weight, tone and lean, increase energy and reach a lower fat percentage.

Eliminate any processed foods, chemicals, artificial sugars, hydrogenated fats and fatty meats. Eat only all natural. Increase protein. Consume little sugar and starch. Drink water at least 6x per day and take a daily probiotic vitamin and electrolyte supplement.

Daily Goal (Food Intake, servings): Greens (3-4), Lean Protein (3-4), Good Carbs (1), Good Fats (2-3), Fruits (2).

MEAL 1

Fruit + Protein

- 1 Cup of fruit (blackberries, blueberries, strawberries) and hardboiled egg
- ½ pink grapefruit, 1 cup low-fat cottage cheese
- ½ cup fruit or ½ banana whipped into 1 cup Greek Yogurt (low-fat, unsweetened)
- 3 slices natural turkey bacon, green apple
- Protein Drink: ½ cup fruit, coconut or spring water, 2 scoops natural protein powder
- ½ cup Sliced Apple, 1 tbsp. raw almond butter, hard boiled egg
- 1 cup fresh fruit, 2 tbsp. wheat germ and ½ cup natural, Greek yogurt (unsweetened).
- 2-4 egg whites, organic turkey bacon (2-4 slices), tomato slices or ½ cup sweet potato home fries

MEAL 2

Good Carb + Fat

- ½ cup rice (short grain brown rice, sprouted jasmine, wild rice) with tsp. oil (extra virgin olive, mct (medium chain triglyceride oil or sunflower oil)
- Brown Rice Cake and tsp. raw nut butter (sunflower, almond, cashew, peanut)
- ½ cup sweet potato or red bliss potatoes (home fries) and tsp. Earth Balance Butter or Coconut Oil
- Slice Ezekiel Toast with 1 tsp natural hummus or avocado and slice tomato
- 1 low-fat mozzarella stick and ½ cup organic carrots
- Brown Rice cake, slice tomato and sprouts
- ½ cup celery or carrot sticks and 1 tsp. avocado or raw almond butter
- ½ cup Ezekiel Almond Cereal with 1 cup nondairy, unsweetened beverage (coconut or almond)
- 1 cup organic sautéed or steamed veggies with tbsp. extra virgin olive oil and 2 ounces lean protein
- 3-4 slices organic deli chicken or turkey slices and 1 cup organic blueberries

MEAL 3

Protein + Veggie + Salad

- 3-5 ounces protein
- 1-2 cups steamed, raw or sautéed veggies in broth
- 1 cup salad greens with fresh squeezed lemon juice
- 1 tbsp. good fat (extra virgin olive oil, mct oil)

Protein (3-6 ounces choices below):

- Light Tuna (in water (wild caught, all natural with no preservatives)
- Fish (wild salmon, shrimp, white fish, scallops)
- Grass Fed, Organic: Chicken Breast, Ground Chicken & Turkey 93% lean, Turkey,
- Grass Fed, Organic: Beef (top round, sirloin, flank), Ground Beef 93% lean
- Tempeh, Tofu
- Egg Whites
- Lentils (1 cup)

*Greens (1-3 Cups choices below):

- Romaine Lettuce
- Baby Kale
- Baby Spinach and Red Spinach
- Arugula
- Red and Green Leaf Lettuce
- Dandelion
- Swiss Chard

*Veggies (1/2 -2 cups choices below):

- Broccoli
- Red Onions
- Beets (roasted)
- Peppers
- Asparagus
- Green Beans
- Carrots
- Tomatoes (fruit)
- Artichoke Hearts
- Asparagus

- o   Edamame
- o   Brussel Sprouts
- o   Cabbage
- o   Cauliflower
- o   Leeks
- o   Celery
- o   Turnips
- o   Zucchini
- o   Cucumber

MEAL 4

FRUIT + PROTEIN

Protein Smoothie

1 cup favorite fruit, 2 scoops natural protein powder and unsweetened organic low-fat milk or nondairy beverage (coconut and/or almond). Blend to taste.

Recommended Proteins:

Orgain Organic Protein Powder (hit link)

MEAL 5

Protein + Greens + Veggie
- 4-6 ounces Protein
- 1 – 2 Cups Greens with Lemon Juice
- ½ Cup Veggies

Or

See below for suggestions.

Clean Dinner Suggestions (fewer the ingredients the better):

- Ground Protein (organic beef, buffalo, chicken or turkey) mixed with sautéed veggies.
- 3-6 ounces White Fish baked in tinfoil with lemon juice, white wine and black pepper. Served with greens and stir fried veggies.
- 3-5 ounces Grilled Free Range Chicken sliced and placed on greens with veggies and Newman's Own Lite Caesar Dressing.
- Ground Protein (organic beef, buffalo, chicken or turkey) mixed with fresh pico de gallo over lettuce and pinch or natural Mexican shredded cheese (Cabot).
- 4-6 ounces Grilled Wild Salmon topped with chopped cucumber, avocado, tomato and lemon juice. Serve with wedge of Pink Grapefruit and salad.
- Scrambled Egg Whites with light cheese and turkey bacon. Two slices tomato and salad with veggies.
- 4-6 ounces Grilled Chicken topped with Bruschetta. Served with steamed asparagus and spinach.
- Organic Bone Broth Chicken Soup with veggies. Served with salad.
- Organic Veggie Broth Soup. Served with quinoa, raw nuts and lentils.
- Tofu sautéed in coconut oil with sliced carrots, chopped onion, garlic clove, cubed sweet potato and seasoning (curry, sea salt and cumin). Served with quinoa, raw nuts and lentils.
- Veggie Chili (lentils, white beans) in a tomato broth with sautéed carrots, onions and peppers. Add tofu or organic ground protein.

Late Night Snack (select one only if needed)

- ½ cup natural Greek Yogurt
- ½ cup natural fruit
- 8 ounce protein drink (8 ounces unsweetened almond milk and Orgain Organic Protein Powder)

Tips:

- ✓ **Cheat Meals & Alcohol:** try to eliminate all for at least 14 days.
- ✓ **Always eat** all natural and whole foods for a long term plan.
- ✓ **Eat smaller** portions.
- ✓ **Make sure lean protein in 3-4 meals**, 3-5 ounces if you are lifting weights.
- ✓ **Eat at home** or know where you'll eat (healthy options).
- ✓ **Stay away from** prepared frozen diet meals at your local supermarket (national brands).
- ✓ **Calories matter** so make sure you try to burn off more than you take in if you're trying to lose weight. Increase activity.
- ✓ **Drink spring water and green tea** (loose leaf) as much as possible.
- ✓ **It's Ok to eat a meal high in fat once in a while.** Eat less and make sure all natural.
- ✓ **Use many** herbs and spices for taste.
- ✓ **If you cheat with a high carb meal. Lift the next day and cut all carbs for that day.**
- ✓ **The Cleaner your foods** the leaner you'll get.
- ✓ **Find 3-4 of your favorite recipes** for protein, veggies and salads. Double the recipe and store for later in the week.
- ✓ **Warm tea and natural seltzer water** can help void cravings.
- ✓ **Food Prep and making sure your fridge and cabinets are stocked** with healthy foods are both key to eating a clean diet.
- ✓ **Track your fitness and calories** with a fitness tracker (i.e. Fitbit)
- ✓ **If you're not losing weight after 3 weeks of dedicated training**. Eliminate all fats for 3-4 days and increase protein along with more cardio. Lift heavier weights and don't get discouraged as you will see progress.

BLEND ALL INGREDIENTS WITH YOUR PREFERED PROTEIN POWDER.
I recommend Orgain Organic Protein Powder as it is smooth, healthy and taste good.

- -
INGREDIENTS
- -

PLAIN JANE

- [x] 1 cup unsweetened vanilla nondairy beverage (coconut, hemp or almond milk # 1 choice)
- [x] 1 tbsp. raw nut butter (almond)
- [x] 2 scoops natural vanilla whey protein plus 2 scoops natural hemp protein
- [x] 1 small semi ripe banana (semi ripe because less sugars)

STRAWBERRY N' BANANA

- [x] 1 cup unsweetened vanilla nondairy beverage (coconut, hemp or almond milk # 1 choice)
- [x] 1 tbsp. raw nut butter (almond)
- [x] 2 scoops natural vanilla whey protein plus 2 scoops natural hemp protein
- [x] 1 tsp. Udo's 3,6,9 blend oil
- [x] ½ cup frozen organic strawberries
- [x] 1 small semi ripe banana (semi ripe because less sugars)

VERY BERRY

- [x] 1 cup unsweetened vanilla nondairy beverage (coconut, hemp or almond milk # 1 choice)
- [x] 1 tbsp. raw nut butter (almond)
- [x] 2 scoops natural vanilla whey protein plus 2 scoops natural hemp protein
- [x] 1 tsp. Udo's 3,6,9 blend oil
- [x] 1 cup organic frozen berry blend (blueberries, raspberries, strawberries)

PINEAPPLE N' BANANA

- [x] 1 cup unsweetened vanilla nondairy beverage (coconut, hemp or almond milk # 1 choice)
- [x] 1 tbsp. raw nut butter (almond)
- [x] 2 scoops natural vanilla whey protein plus 2 scoops natural hemp protein
- [x] 1 tsp. Udo's 3,6,9 blend oil
- [x] 1 small semi ripe banana
- [x] ½ cup frozen or naturally canned pineapple in juice

CHOCOLATE N' STRAWBERRY

- [x] 1 cup unsweetened chocolate nondairy beverage (coconut, hemp or almond milk # 1 choice)
- [x] 1 tbsp. raw nut butter (almond)
- [x] 2 scoops chocolate whey protein plus 2scoops natural hemp protein
- [x] 1 tsp. Udo's 3,6,9 blend oil
- [x] ½ cup frozen organic strawberries

AFTERWORD

Well that's it for **the Upper Body Reboot Fix**. I hope you will try your best and stick to the program as closely as possible. The key to losing weight and great results is making mindful food choices and training with intensity based upon your fitness level. Always try to live by the rule of, "You are what you eat!" If you eat healthy, you'll be healthy. Simple, as that. Of course, exercise is a key component, but nutrition is the main factor to looking fit and faster results. By the way, if you have any questions or concerns related to this or any of your fitness concerns. Please email me, Doug Bennett, at bsstudio@comcast.net Title the subject line, "Body Reboot Series ". For extra diet, fitness information and tips...visit www.fitactions.com

Simply, add your name and email to get more FREE workouts and tips to get into the best shape of your life. Don't Forget to check out our Social Sites for FREE VIDEOS, TIPS and RECIPES:

Instagram: www.instagram.com/Toptrainersworkouts
Facebook: www.facebook.com/gogirlfit

YouTube: The Bennett Method https://www.youtube.com/user/fitgy321

Other Books and Programs:

Amazon:
21 Day Total Body Tone Up Guide: A Complete At-Home 21-Day Plan To Get You Lean, Strong, Fit and Looking Hot, FAST!
The 42 Day Lower Body Fix

Apple IApps:
Fitgirl Pro
15 Minute Metabolic Burners

Made in United States
North Haven, CT
21 May 2022